Happy Healing!

Asa Roberts

The Cancer Journal ~ Heal Yourself!

How To Cure Cancer Series

10 Key Principles Others Use To Cure Themselves
Recipes For Amazing Herbal Medicines Proven To
Kill Cancer
Expert Nutrition Advice, Tips and Warnings
Empowering Information That Will Change Your
Beliefs About Cancer Forever . . .

and much, much more . . .

Lisa Robbins

the good witch publishing

Ontario, Canada

The Cancer Journal ~ Heal Yourself!
How To Cure Cancer Series

the good witch publishing

Ontario, Canada
Orders @ http://thegoodwitch.ca/cauldron_shop/

Bulk Orders Send Email to tgw@TheGoodWitch.ca

Editor: Thank You! Mary McGillis, Author and Celtic Storyteller ~
Infusing Our World with Ancient Spiritual Knowing.
www.MaryMcGillis.com

Technical Editing Advice: Thank You! Judi Peers, Author

Cover Design: Thank You! Paul Clark, WAVE
www.WeAreVirtuallyEverywhere.com

International Standard Book Numbers

Softcover   **978-0-9864902-2-4**

Electronic Book   978-0-9864902-1-7
Audiobook   978-0-9864902-3-1

REVIEWS

"I wish my father had this information 12 years ago. You're gonna save a lot of lives Lisa!! Amazing book!!"
Tyler Davis

~~~

"Hi Lisa, read your book yesterday and was amazed with the information. Will buy a copy for everyone in my family. Like you, both my parents died of cancer, my Father had it twice in fact. Anyway, wanted you to know that I am blown away with what you have achieved and you should be proud, I know your parents would be."
Lynn Hill, President MultiLink Business Management Solutions

~~~

"I have read about many types of alternative and integrative treatments for cancer. I have read your book and absolutely love it. It is one of my favorites so far."
Iliana Dedona

~~~

"The Cancer Journal ~ Heal Yourself was written by Lisa Robbins over the course of 10 years, and absolutely is one of the greatest gifts we will ever know. Lisa documents losing both of her parents to the standard North American tortuous cancer treatments, and her ensuing journey to the discovery that cancer has already been beaten. The CAnswer is in her must read book ~ in a story so compelling and simple that each and every one of us owes it to our ourselves, to our ancestors and to our children to read the book now. Like many of us, I have lost family to cancer, but now know that this disease can be a part of our history, if we all would only act on what Lisa has taught. Learn the 10 key principles of healing, learn how to make anti-cancer teas, learn about tragedies that didn't have to be. Get ready to cry and laugh and then to really live.
Thank you LISA ROBBINS aka The Good Witch!"
Mary McGillis, Author of *Hector and The Little People* and Editor of *The Cancer Journal ~ Heal Yourself!*

Table of Contents

Dedications

This journal is dedicated to:

My mother, Doris Elisabeth, who battled cancer and the effects of surgeries and treatments until she died in palliative care on December 9, 2007; and to my father, Ronald William who battled cancer, treatments and surgeries, until a huge dose of chemotherapy ravaged his already sick and weakened body and caused him to die on October 18, 1987, at the age of 54;

My husband Bob for putting up with my obsession, my daughter Alix for inspiring me to take TheGoodWitch to the highest level, my son Luke for doing all the house repairs and renovations as I write, and my daughter Anna for making me thousands of cups of tea and encouraging me to work my fingers to the bone;

Harry Hoxsey, Rene Caisse, the Hamilton boy, Daniel Hauser, Pattie MacDonald, Linda Devine, Jay Kordich, Kerri Howarth, Yvonne Chamberlain, Greg Caton, Dr. Gustavo Bounous, Billy Best and John Robbins for their incredible contributions to our world of healing naturally;

All those who have fought their own brave battle with cancer and lost, to those suffering the ravages of cancer now and to those whose cancer diagnosis is yet to come;

May the truth now and forever set you free . . .

Disclaimer

Would you like to interact with the electronic version of The Cancer Journal ~ Heal Yourself!?

If you are reading the printed copy of this book and you would like to be able to click on the links provided and be taken to the articles, videos, audios, transcripts, studies, recipes, databases and essential resources, send us a copy of your receipt for this book and we will give you a link to access the interactive electronic copy free of charge. Send your receipt to contact@thegoodwitch.ca with '**send my free copy**' in the subject line.

We reserve the right to discontinue this offer at any time.

Intentions

The following intentions have been embedded throughout this journal:

- To unite our beliefs about healing naturally so you can wholly embrace the ideas and techniques used and feel comfortable and knowledgeable in this practice;

- To empower you to *heal yourself* by connecting you to the stories of how others have healed themselves with safe and effective natural methods;

- To bring medicinal plants into your kitchen, so you can quickly and easily prepare effective herbal medicines and benefit from their miraculous healing properties anytime you need to;

- To teach you simple techniques that make eating nutritious and delicious healing foods part of your everyday life;

- To impart essential knowledge about your body and the environment in which your health flourishes and disease is nonexistent;

- To connect you with resources for further study and research so you may quickly become an expert in the areas that are relevant and important to you.

Imagine Our World Without Cancer . . .

Can you? Yes . . . you can!

There is a collective movement that is quietly seeping into the stronghold of the cancer establishment. It is a powerful movement of educated and intelligent people, the healers and the healed, working together to share their messages of hope and health.

In this journal you will meet Linda Devine, a courageous woman who refused conventional medical treatment for breast cancer and cured herself with diet and lifestyle changes within ten months. No tumor, no cancer. No surgery, no radiation. You will meet others who have refused conventional treatments and gone on to heal themselves. Their triumphant stories of curing cancer by using simple, natural methods are the catalyst for changing our world of cancer, from one of devastation and disease to one of hope and healing.

Since the early 1900s, the medical establishment has used political ties to influence laws that create a monopoly on cancer treatments. The industry has used underhanded marketing tactics, based on our most primitive of emotions, fear, to create a multibillion dollar industry that supports the tortuous and inhumane treatments used in conventional cancer centers right now.

Over those 100 years, and for many years before, certain knowledgeable people have spent their lives quietly curing cancer with safe, natural methods.

Why then do people continue to trudge day after day into oncology units across Canada, the United States and around the world, to subject themselves to toxic and tortuous treatments?

Unfortunately, most people believe that the conventional way is the only way.

The fact remains: Thousands have healed themselves by using nutritional, herbal and alternative therapies and many more continue to do so.

When I was twenty years old and my father was undergoing cancer treatments, I found a small lump on my leg. I was sure I was going to die and could think of nothing else until a doctor convinced me that it was a small muscle abnormality.

Last year an old friend was diagnosed with a cancerous tumor on her leg. She was so terrified by the diagnosis, before having a CT Scan, she vomited and drove two hours back to her home town to rest. Only then could she gather the courage to go back for the test.

As I sit here writing this introduction, I am wrought with anguish as I realize how much we are caught up in the fear created and nurtured by the conventional cancer industry.

Natural cleansing and supportive nutrition and lifestyle practices are the only terms under which nature provides a *cure* for cancer.

Until we embrace our connection with our earth's natural foods and medicines and truly realize and accept our own innate ability to heal; we will continue to harm ourselves with ridiculous treatments that destroy our body's defenses and allow cancer to grow more prolifically than before.

Chemotherapy causes cancer. Radiation causes cancer. Diagnostic tools using radiation, such as CT scans and bone scans, cause cancer. Even mammograms have been added to the long list of current medical practices that cause damage and increase your risks of getting cancer.

Herbal medicines, juicing, cleansing, super nutrition, proper sun exposure, rest; these are things that prevent and cure cancer. Finally, there is enough information and experiential evidence to propel us forward into a world without cancer.

Lisa Robbins, BScHN, RHN, CTT

To the point of no return . . .

"

All truths are easy to understand once they are discovered; the point is to discover them.

"

Galileo Galilei

1 Indoctrination

Cancer.

No other word evokes more fear.

Certainly for my family, the word cancer generates not only fear, but memories of tragic loss and suffering.

It is 1978 and we are living a dream. My father is working for Digital Equipment Corporation in Galway, Ireland. We moved from Canada only seven months before. On his days off we gallivant around the Irish countryside in a tiny Fiat, soaking in Irish culture and honing our Gaelic accents. We stand at the edge of the beautiful Cliffs of Moher, breathing in the fresh, wafting smell of the sea. We happily eat thick, brown Irish soda bread, dipped in spicy mussel soup at Dirty Nelly's, our family's favorite Irish pub.

I am eighteen and sublimely ignorant about cancer.

Fast forward two years. In the fall, my father becomes ill and is admitted to an Irish hospital. Doctors find a large tumor sitting tightly flush with his right kidney. He is immediately flown home to Canada, where surgeons remove the tumor, along with his right kidney and spleen.

Back in 1974, we were living in Timmins, Ontario, where my father was working for Senator Motor Hotels. My mother and father had a serious misunderstanding, an argument that caused my mother to find refuge in Toronto with her relatives. During this one-week period, my father scrambled to do something that would impress my mother on her return. He chose to strip and re-wax all the floors in our home. He used industrial strength floor stripper and wax from the hotel. I remember him proudly standing in front of our shiny, clean floors on her return. She was so happy that he had gone to such trouble to apologize.

My father wasn't feeling well after his gallant effort and over the next few days he became terribly ill, the whites of his eyes turning a nasty yellow. He was admitted to the hospital in Timmins, diagnosed with hepatitis. His liver had suffered damage from the strong industrial floor stripper. Over the next few weeks, my father slowly recovered and life returned to normal.

Other situations contributed to my father's illness; like two stomach ulcers, both times doctors removed large parts of his stomach. In the 1970s, although scientists knew most stomach ulcers in pigs were caused by the bacterium Heliobacter Pylori, we had not applied this knowledge to humans. Instead of a simple antibiotic regimen that is common today, my father suffered through two stomach surgeries which left him unable to properly digest his food or absorb the nutrients he so desperately needed.

My mother was a fantastic cook and we ate healthy meals at home, but because of his job, my father ate at restaurants all the time. Stress, alcohol and cigarettes were a large part of his life. He ate hot dogs and bacon on a regular basis and drank big glasses of homogenized cow's milk every day, all contributors to my father's ill health, poor immunity and emergence of tumors . . .

"

Thinking back . . .

I visit my father in Toronto General Hospital. It is devastating. He seems barely alive. Machines are everywhere, tubes are running in and out of his body, delivering medication and taking away bodily fluids. We are all in shock.

The surgeon says my father will not live long, but they will keep him on morphine until he dies, maybe four months. The surgeon turns out to be very wrong.

Soon after his surgery, doctors want to *make sure no cancer is left*. They radiate the area where they removed his kidney and spleen, without allowing the underlying tissues time to heal. His suffering increases exponentially. For two and a half years afterward, the wound cannot heal and continually festers, with internal stitches appearing one by one in a bubbling vat of infection.

We begin to wonder if his doctors *really* know what they are doing.

Over the next nine years, my father suffers unbelievably. The radiation makes him sick and weak. He can only eat small amounts of food. He loses close to one-hundred pounds. He is regularly nauseated and always tired, very tired. His quality of life is nonexistent. It is too painful to watch.

Finally in the fall of 1987, doctors make a last ditch effort to *save* him. They blast him with chemotherapy. As sick as he already is, they kick him while he is down. The chemotherapy literally kills him. He cannot eat and can barely speak as yeast takes over his body and his mouth and throat fill with white pustules of infection. His ankles lose their definition from swelling as his kidney function deteriorates. His blood pressure falls dangerously low and his damaged heart can no longer pump blood through his arteries.

He succumbs and dies in Princess Margaret Hospital on October 18, 1987. He is only 54 years old. We are relieved when his suffering ends . . . so is he.

I am eight months pregnant with my first child. Sadly, my father misses meeting his new baby granddaughter by thirty-four days. I can feel him every time I look into her beautiful, blue eyes.

I flatly declare that the usual hospital treatment today, in a case of tumorous growth, most certainly leads to worsening of the disease, or a speedier death, and in healthy people, quickly causes cancer.

Johanna Budwig, 1994, Seven Time Nobel Prize Nominee.

3

2   A Living Nightmare

After my father dies I am too busy raising children to think much about what has happened. It isn't until my mother is diagnosed with cancer in 1999, that I really become desperate to find a solution to my family's cancer problems.

She visits her family physician for an annual breast exam and has prepared a list of questions. She has been feeling tired and ill and can feel a lump in her abdomen on the lower left side. As he is examining her breast she asks him about it. "It's just a stool," he tells her.

When the examination is complete, she brings the list of questions from her purse and begins asking the doctor. He immediately gets angry and says, "I don't have time for this. You have to make another appointment." He leaves the room.

For other reasons, as well as her physician's obvious disregard for her health, she never returns for more of his advice. She looks for two years for another doctor, but no physician in this area is taking patients. Thousands of people are without doctors.

During the summer, her skin begins to turn a sickly grey color. She is obviously very ill and we urge her to see another doctor.

My sister-in-law pleads with her physician to take my mother on as a patient. He agrees and sees my mother. He immediately orders an x-ray and finds a tumor the size of a mandarin orange, growing through the wall of her bowel. She is diagnosed with Dukes C adenocarcinoma of the colon.

She needs transfused blood before she can have surgery; she has lost so much blood from the tumor site. She is tired and deathly anemic.

Doctors remove the tumor and resection her colon. Cancer cells are found in two of four extracted lymph nodes.

Cancer is rooted in every drop of blood in the body and we may as well expect to stop the growing of apples by picking them off trees, or to stop the springing of dandelions by cutting off the blossoms and leaving the root in the ground, as to expect to destroy malignancy in the human body by attacking the outward growth.

Dr. Robert Bell, *Cancer is a Blood Disease and Must Be Treated as Such,* New York Medical Record, March 18, 1922.

3   What Is Cancer?

It is the summer of 1999 and I begin to read all I can get my hands on about cancer. The library has practically nothing. All the publications in the hospital only tell patients how to deal with the side effects of their treatments.

I am working at a nursing college, which gives me access to medical and nursing journals.

I begin saving, sorting and filing hundreds of documents about cancer, articles, reports, studies, brochures, contacts and advertising pieces.

Research shows that all animals can get cancer and even plants develop cancers. Crown gall is a form of plant cancer.

Cancer occurs when a cell or cells have become damaged by: chemical pollutants, toxins, synthetic hormones, viruses, parasites, excessive heat or cold, or radiation. Damaged cells can no longer protect themselves and fungi and other pathogens move into the cell, releasing hormones, toxins and wastes, damaging DNA and disrupting the cell's ability to function normally.

Tumors are not foreign; they arise from the same tissues that make up our bodies, but several factors must be in place for a tumor to form. We'll talk more about these later.

Cancer can grow in your brain, bones, muscles, blood, cells and organs, anywhere really. It pops up rather like mold pops up on leftovers in the refrigerator.

I always imagine a puffball when I think of tumors. Puffballs are very large, egg-shaped, edible mushrooms. They arise on the forest floor almost instantaneously. One day there is no hint of a puffball, then all of a sudden they appear. Puffballs seem to mature just as fast as they appear. If you wait too long to pick a puffball, it will turn to dust when you touch it, spreading millions of spores in all directions. Fungi . . . tumor like . . .

We have been taught that exposure to mutagenic or carcinogenic compounds damages the portion of DNA which programs apoptosis or cell death, creating a process of unlimited growth. In other words, chemicals and radiation create mutant genes through their ability to damage DNA. The cell now grows out of control forming a mass or tumor.

However, this is not exactly the way cancer forms and this is not exactly what cancer really is, as you will soon find out . . .

Cancer – latin karkinos, the crab . . . malignant neoplasia, marked by uncontrolled growth of cells.

Malignant – growing worse, resisting treatment, harmful, tending or threatening to produce death.

Neoplasia – development of neoplasms, new and abnormal formation of tissue, with no useful function, grows at expense of healthy organism.

Venes & Thomas, *Taber's Cyclopedic Medical Dictionary*, 2001.

4   Diet and Cancer

I begin to study holistic nutrition and learn about the powerful effects of natural phytochemicals from food, what individual symptoms and patterns of symptoms mean and about using foods and medicinal herbs by themselves or in balanced combinations to nourish and heal.

Fresh, raw, organic, whole foods and herbs carry nutrients which your body uses to protect and heal itself. Meals prepared with traditional methods preserve valuable nutrients in fresh foods and in some cases add to the nutritional value, as in fermentation of sauerkraut, yogurt, miso, brined pickles and tempeh. Traditional cultures use foods that have a natural way of protecting us from all types of disease, including cancer.

Without proper nutrition, your immune cells cannot proliferate adequately, your cells cannot produce antioxidants to protect themselves and your body lacks defense against cancer and other diseases. Nutrition matters so much that without it, you cannot expect to rebuild your body, so that it may fight disease for you. With what, would your cells manufacture glutathione, their protective antioxidant, if they didn't have the key essential components with which to build it?

When nutrition is functional, as in traditional diets, disease simply does not happen.

During the early 1900s, Dr. Weston Price toured the world with a camera and notepad and recorded the results of his study into the relationship between nutrition and dental decay. What Dr. Price made note of was a direct correlation between what we eat and how healthy we are.

In the tribes he studied, traditional diets rich in whole, natural foods grew healthy people with no dental cavities. Foods most prized include eggs, liver, whole milk and butter, bone broths, cod liver oil and seafood. No modern convenience foods with high amounts of sugars and additives. No synthetic supplements. No hydrogenated or partially hydrogenated fats.

When people from these tribes were raised in areas where processed foods were available, they had nutrient deficiencies and ate more chemicals and added sugars. Not only did their teeth decay but their facial bones formed improperly causing their teeth to crowd. They had lower IQ's, more personality disturbances and higher rates of disease (Ballentine, 1978).

I start to learn that the relationship between what we eat and cancer is more important than anything else.

I am one of millions of people who have been inspired by the writing of John Robbins. His book, *A Diet For A New America: How Your Food Choices Affect Your Health, Happiness, and the Future of Life on Earth*, made me want to be a vegetarian more than any other book I have read.

John's message is clear. Stop eating animals and their milk, for moral reasons as well as the amazing health benefits you will feel when you replace high protein, fat-laden foods with nourishing, whole plant foods.

John analyzes hundreds of studies to compile enormous proof of the disease-causing effects of a diet based on meat and dairy foods and the benefits of eating a plant-centered diet. He dispels the myths about humans requiring high amounts of protein and calcium from meat and dairy foods.

This book woke me up to the plight of feed and dairy animals. They are not the happy-looking chicken on a package of processed chicken loaf, or the contented, smiling cow on the milk carton, that is used to feed milk to children at schools, in a milk campaign, sponsored by the Milk Board . . . They are helpless, intelligent animals that we disrespect, abuse and then eat. We cause them to feel hopelessness, disgust and finally terror; the reality of which, we have been completely distanced from (Robbins, 1987).

The Healthiest People On Earth

What if we could study the eating habits of the healthiest people on earth?

In *Healthy at 100: How You Can – At Any Age – Dramatically Increase Your Life Span and Your Health Span*, John Robbins has compiled an in-depth analysis of the eating and lifestyle habits of cultures in different parts of the world, whose populations are high in centenarians – those who live one-hundred years or more.

John explains that elders from Hunza, Okinawa, Abkhasia and Vilcabamba have 'retained their faculties, remained vigorous, and enjoyed life right up until only weeks or months before their deaths.' He states that elders from these traditional populations have extremely low rates of degenerative diseases such as cancer, heart disease, arthritis and dementia and that they remain unusually fit and active throughout their lifetimes.

What is the diet of the Hunzakuts, Okinawans, Abkhasians and Vilcabambans?

9

You might guess it is based on fresh picked, mostly raw, vegetables, fruits, nuts, seeds, whole grains, legumes, tiny amounts of fermented dairy and very little or no meat.

Their diets have very little saturated fat, no trans fats, no pasteurized (cooked) dairy, no sugar, fried foods, chemicals, hormones or additives – no foods that take profuse amounts of digestive enzymes to process, no foods that form acids, congest your body with toxic buildup and cause degenerative disease (Robbins, 2006).

I soon learn from following my parents through the disease process that the information they desperately need to heal themselves is being deliberately kept from them.

Nutrition Advice From The Oncology Department

The only nutrition advice given to my mother is how to eat more food when she does not feel like eating at all because she is so sick from toxic chemotherapy treatments. My mother is given a brochure called 'Living Well With Cancer,' which includes several fact sheets about cancer. I hope it includes information on how to eat properly. Unbelievably the *expert* advice on the fact sheet on 'Healthy Eating' tells my mother, "Everyone should eat healthy food. This is especially true for people with cancer."

The focus of the brochure is to promote eating foods, "high in protein and calories before, during, and after treatment." The foods suggested are, "eggs, cheese, dairy products, cold meats, nuts, tofu and dried peas and beans." The brochure goes on to say, "healthy foods high in calories include muffins, puddings, cookies, dried fruit, granola and sandwiches" (Healthy Eating Brochure, 2001).

What does this information tell my mother? To eat muffins, puddings, cookies, granola, sandwiches, cheese, dairy and cold meats? These are the very foods that contributed to her problems in the first place!

The 'Healthy Eating' fact sheet tells my mother to follow Canada's Food Guide, again which places focus on foods that are difficult to digest and assimilate, like cooked cold meat and cheese. There is no mention of eating raw food, which maximizes nutritional assimilation. Nothing about increasing immune stimulating raw garlic and onions or highly unsaturated cancer fighting fats. It does not warn about high sugar levels and encourages my mother to eat up to ten grains per day. Ten grains per day would cause a bucketload of problems for most people, especially those with cancer, and specifically for my mother who only has half of her stomach left, after two stomach surgeries for ulcers!

10

The other fact sheets have nothing to do with helping my mother overcome cancer. They ironically have pictures of calming clouds and happy people. They ALL are designed to prepare her for the debilitating and tortuous treatments she is about to receive.

The other fact sheets given to *help* my mother are entitled:
Pain
Radiation Therapy
Understanding Medical Words
Fatigue
Anemia
Nausea and Vomiting
Hair Loss
Surgery
Combination Therapy
(Surgery, chemotherapy and
radiation used in various
combinations)
Choosing Your Central Venous Access Devices
Chemotherapy

Sounds a lot like a word cloud of devastation. Where is the hope? Where is the real information about cancer and all the natural foods and herbs that fight it?

I notice the group who distribute the 'Healthy Living' fact sheets. From the 'Living Well With Cancer' sheets, "Living Well With Cancer is a partnership among people living with cancer, health care professionals, people who represent cancer and professional organizations, and Ortho Biotech" (Living Well With Cancer, 2010). Ortho Biotech is a pharmaceutical company making products for the cancer industry.

One piece of information suggests my mother see an Oncology Dietician, but this information is not designed to help her overcome cancer either. It states the Oncology Dietician provides nutrition advice to patients to help them maintain *adequate nourishment* during treatments. They emphasize that making the right choices about which foods to eat, can prevent, control and reverse some side effects of treatment. These side effects include nausea and vomiting, diarrhea, constipation, sore mouth and throat, loss of appetite, weight loss, swallowing problems, taste changes and weight gain (Living Well With Cancer, 2010).

Report – Food, Nutrition and the Prevention of Cancer
In 1997 and again in 2007, the World Cancer Research Fund and the American Institute of Cancer Research brought together a panel of experts from twenty countries, to examine the available evidence on the

11

relationship between diet and cancer. The review entitled 'Food, Nutrition and the Prevention of Cancer: A Global Perspective,' concludes the following: Lacto-ovo, lacto-vegetarian and vegan diets provide decreased risk for colon, breast and prostate cancer. The panel concluded the exclusion of meat and inclusion of a variety of plant foods was likely responsible for decreased cancer risk. Experts state:

The capacity of a cell to achieve effective cancer prevention or REPAIR is dependent on the extracellular microenvironment, including the availability of energy and the presence of appropriate macro and micro nutrients . . .

'Food, Nutrition and the Prevention of Cancer: A Global Perspective,' 2007.

My emphasis on *repair*.

The report summarizes the following recommendations:
1. Be as lean as possible, within the normal range of body weight.
2. Be physically active as part of everyday life.
3. Limit consumption of energy dense foods and avoid sugary drinks.
4. East mostly foods of plant origin.
5. Limit intake of red meat and avoid processed meat.
6. Limit alcoholic drinks.
7. Limit consumption of salt and avoid moldy grains and legumes.
8. Aim to meet nutritional needs through diet alone.
9. Mothers to breastfeed; children to be breastfed exclusively for six months.
10. Follow the recommendations for cancer prevention: All cancer survivors to receive **nutritional care** from an appropriately trained professional (World Cancer Research Fund, 2007).

My emphasis on *nutritional care*.

Energy Restriction fights cancer
Interestingly, the report shows that, 'restriction of energy intake from food is the most effective single intervention' for preventing cancer in experimental animals! (World Cancer Research Fund, 2007).

For centuries we have known that fasting improves our health. Many groups still use fasting today as a way to improve their health and

12

connect spiritually; moving toward a more enlightened, happy and contented way of living.

Through elimination of built up wastes and toxins, fasting provides clarity of mind, increased energy, weight loss and improved function of every cell, tissue and organ in your body. We will talk about fasting in more detail soon.

I often observe in fasting participants that concentration improves, creative thinking expands, depression lifts, insomnia ceases, anxieties fade, minds become more tranquil, and the natural joy of living begins to reappear. It is my hypothesis that when the physical toxins are cleared from the brain cells, mind-brain function automatically and significantly improves, and spiritual capacities expand.

Gabriel Cousens, 2010.

5 Chemotherapy, Radiation & Second Cancers

I am in the Oncology Department of the hospital with my mother. It's a very disheartening place to be. Everywhere there are deathly ill people with no hair, no energy, no life. I feel like I'm in hell with them. My mother's oncologist has an accent and I can't help but think of him as 'Dr. Hitler.' He offers her a chance to be in a study of new chemotherapy drugs. Half the patients will receive a new drug, the other half will receive the old drug. She painfully worries that she may not get the new drug, as if it has a secret advantage over the old one, some magic way of killing cancer cells without killing her.

Chemotherapy is chemotherapy. All forms of it are poisonous and carcinogenic. Imagine the treatment for cancer causing cancer. It is so ironic and too heinous to believe ...

After all, and for the overwhelming majority of the cases, there is no proof whatsoever that chemotherapy prolongs survival expectations. And this is the great lie about this therapy, that there is a correlation between the reduction of cancer and the extension of the life of the patient.

Phillip Day, 1999.

During our first meeting I am so wound up I cannot sit down. 'Dr. Hitler' gets visibly disturbed and asks me to sit down three times. I do not oblige and this makes him defensive. I ask him if he can assure my mother that if she decides to accept his only treatment option, chemotherapy, that it will most certainly not increase her risk for other cancers.

He says the only thing he can say, "No, I can't assure you of that."

How ironic is it that the oath physicians recite on indoctrination into medical society is, 'Do no harm.' No natural therapist would ever order chemotherapy for her clients. All natural therapists are taught to use

14

effective, health-supporting, natural therapies, to improve the body's ability to fight disease.

Unfortunately, Canadian and U.S. health laws prohibit natural therapists from saving cancer patients. Instead, patients are coerced into being poisoned with chemotherapy and radiation, all the time believing this is the only way. How horrifically sad and unnecessary.

With seven chemotherapy treatments over two months, my mother becomes extremely ill and her doctor has to write a discontinue order. He orders blood transfusions to clear some of the poison from her system. She weighs only 108 pounds and is deathly ill.

I find myself wondering if Dr. Hitler would take the drug himself.

After four days of rest and care, being fed only fresh, raw carrot juice, mixed raw vegetable juices, and homemade soups; she is feeling better and is ready to go back to her own home.

Several months later in 2000, a CT scan finds two small tumors in her right lung. Later I realize that this is a major turning point for my mother. At sixty-six years old, she has surgery to remove the lung tumors.

SECOND CANCERS CAUSED DIRECTLY BY TREATMENTS

I call the Canadian Cancer Society's Information Service. I ask the 'Cancer Information Specialist' for information on chemotherapy and radiation causing second cancers. She says she is also interested in this information. Three weeks later, she sends me links to two studies.

An article from the American Cancer Society's website, 'Second Cancers Caused by Cancer Treatment' reports that several Leukemias have been linked to previous radiation exposure: *Acute myelogenous leukemia (AML), chronic myelogenous leukemia (CML), and acute lymphoblastic leukemia.*

Chemotherapy causes Leukemia faster than Radiation therapy. Patients treated in the seventies and eighties for Hodgkin disease, non-Hodgkins lymphoma, ovarian cancer, lung cancer and breast cancer have increased risk for Acute myelogenous leukemia. (American Cancer Society, 2009).

The thoracic surgeon cuts her breastbone down the middle, pulls her ribs apart and excises nine small tumors in total. He tells us he felt her lung all over with his hands to find the tumors in her right lung and he used the same process on her left lung but did not find any tumors there.

Her dinner tray comes the day after her surgery. It looks like dog food. Some kind of frozen meat patty, canned corn and fake mashed potatoes. Her dessert is peaches from a can. I am disgusted. How can they feed garbage like this to sick people? No nutrition whatsoever. It is *almost* like they do not want people to get better. Isn't a hospital a place where people are supposed to heal?

Her recovery is brutal. She can't even get out of bed for weeks. The surgery is way too stressful on her body and she takes months to recover. Truthfully, she never really does recover. The surgery does not help the tumor in her right bronchi. Shortly after the surgery and for the next seven years when the constant coughing becomes too much, she agrees to have the tumor cut out with a metal tube or burned with a laser to free her airway.

Several full-time scientists at the McGill Cancer Center sent to 118 doctors, all experts on lung cancer, a questionnaire to determine the level of trust they had in the therapies they were applying; they were asked to imagine that they themselves had contracted the disease and which of the six current experimental therapies they would choose. Seventy nine doctors answered, 64 of them said that they would not consent to undergo any treatment containing cis-platinum – one of the common chemotherapy drugs they used – while 58 out of 79 believed that all the experimental therapies above were not accepted because of the ineffectiveness and the elevated level of toxicity of chemotherapy.

Phillip Day, 1999.

SECOND CANCERS CAUSED DIRECTLY BY TREATMENTS

The second article is entitled, 'Can Radiation Therapy Influence the Development of Second Cancers?'

It is posted on the National Cancer Institute's site. The article states that radiotherapy and chemotherapy may be a contributing factor for some people to develop a completely new primary cancer (National Cancer Institute, 2007).

6   Cancer Prevention and Politics

I register for a course entitled *Cancer Prevention and Politics*. I have never seen those two words in one sentence, but I feel their *malignant* connection every time I accompany my mother to a doctor's appointment.

I dive into the material and text for the *Cancer Prevention and Politics* course. This is exactly what I have been looking for. The course text is called *When Healing Becomes A Crime* by Kenny Ausubel. It's a thorough work on the life of naturopathic doctor and cancer healer, Harry Hoxsey. The book completely changes the way I think about cancer and the conventional cancer community forever. I become understandably skeptical about anything they say and do.

Hoxsey's life (1901 to 1974) is an amazing story of triumph over cancer even in the face of devious repression, coercion and manipulation by FDA and government officials. If you have ever doubted the suppression of cancer cures, Ausubel's account will forever change your mind.

What was so special about Hoxsey's therapies that certain high ranking government and FDA officials tried desperately to suppress them? Hoxsey's therapies cured thousands of people, with many different types of cancer. From the famous story of nurse Mildred Nelson's mother, severely burned from radiation treatments for uterine cancer, and left for dead by her doctors, to an elderly farmer cured of a huge cancer on the top of his head . . . Hoxsey's therapies saved lives!

The baby of thirteen children, Harry Hoxsey came to own the largest cancer clinic in the world in the 1950s. In 1957, the Hoxsey Clinic had seven physicians, twenty-six nurses, eight x-ray technicians (for diagnosis only), and five laboratory technicians. Patients attended the clinic from all over the world and the clinic served about 150 new patients per week. Thousands of patients swore that Harry Hoxsey's treatment cured them (Ausubel, 2000).

There were three formulas. One was a tonic or tea which could be taken internally. One was a caustic red paste, which killed anything it was applied to, including healthy flesh. The third remedy was a yellow powder, which reportedly killed only malignant tissue (Hoxsey, 1957).

Harry claimed an 80 percent cure rate, and his remedies are known today to be *the most effective* of all the natural remedies for cancer. Harry was repeatedly hounded by the AMA, the FDA and the NCI (National Cancer Institute). In a two year period he was arrested over 100 times (Ausubel, 2000).

A Dallas judge in federal court attested to the efficacy of Hoxsey's treatments:

Hoxsey's therapy is comparable to surgery, radium and x-ray in its effectiveness, without the destructive side effects of those treatments.

Ausubel, 2000.

Hoxsey therapies were upheld by a team of physicians who inspected his Dallas clinic in 1954 and concluded that Hoxsey's clinic was successfully treating internal and external cancers, without surgery, radium or x-ray. The 1950s had not yet seen the widespread use of chemotherapy. The American Medical Association and the Food and Drug Administration admitted that his treatment could cure some forms of cancer (Ausubel, 2000).

Harry repeatedly tried to get the AMA, FDA and NCI to test his formulas against their treatments. Just as many times as he asked, they refused. In 1960, the AMA finally succeeded in driving Hoxsey's therapies out of the U.S. and banned the sale of his medications (Ausubel, 2000).

During the 1960s many doctors were using a paste identical to Harry Hoxsey's original medicine. They reported cancers of the nose, outer ear and other organs, completely healed. The Bio-Medical Center in Mexico, run by Mildred Nelson, Hoxsey's dedicated nurse for years, until her death in 1999 retains records that report complete healings of many patients, even some with late stage disease. According to Ausubel, Hoxsey's therapy consisted of an herbal tonic, diet modifications, vitamin and mineral supplements and counseling (Ausubel, 2000).

The Bio-Medical Center continues to cure cancer with Hoxsey's original formulas and diet therapy. When Yvonne Chamberlain decided to heal herself naturally, twenty-eight years ago, she left Australia and her young family and travelled halfway across the world to stay at the Bio-Medical Center in Mexico. They applied a paste to her deadly black melanoma, and in ten days it fell completely off. The Bio-Medical Center, P.O. Box 727, 615 General Ferreira, Colonia juarez, Tijuana, B.C. Mexico. Telephone 52-814-9011.

Some of the most *effective* scientists and healers have spent their entire lives combining a passion for helping people with tested, natural methods for eradicating cancer. Oddly enough, every time natural healers try to apply their proven techniques to help others in the fight against cancer, they and their therapies are suppressed.

Why do you suppose that is?

I suppose it's because we are being manipulated. Not only are we being manipulated, we are also being mutilated, maimed and murdered.

The clinic is successfully treating pathologically proven cases of cancer, both internal and external, without surgery, radium or x-ray.

Team of Physicians who examined Hoxsey's clinic in 1954. Ausubel, 2000.

7 Money and Greed

Just the other day, I received a fold-out brochure from the Princess Margaret Hospital in Toronto, the place where my father received his fatal chemotherapy injections, and my mother received her debilitating radiation treatments. They have changed their slogan to be, "Conquer Cancer In Our Lifetime."

They want me to donate money to their *cause* . . .

The huge, *profitable,* non-profit and not-for-profit companies, medical societies, pharmaceutical giants and certain high-ranking government officials, with financial ties to these organizations, are continuing to suppress herbal and nutritional therapies for the self-serving goal of protecting their financial interests.

Straight up, their main focus is profit. Natural therapies cannot be patented; so they are not profitable enough.

I know you have heard this before.

Why would corporate giants invest time and money in an herbal therapy that costs $50 for six months, when they make *billions* pushing present treatments?

Why would they promote natural healing when synthetic treatments are so lucrative?

Becoming educated about cancer and the politics surrounding it has been the best thing I could *ever* have done to protect myself and my family.

Fundraising For The Cancer Industry
I use mostly Canadian statistics below but the gist of this information applies anywhere, including The United States and European countries.

In the fiscal year ended January 2009, The Canadian Cancer Society's Ontario Division, showed revenues of $112,178,000. This income came from a variety of sources including individual and corporate giving and planned fundraising activities (Canada Revenue Agency, 2010).

The Canadian Cancer Society's 'Annual Report' shows revenue of $220,151,000, for fiscal year ended January 31, 2010. This shows combined income last year for all thirteen divisions of the Canadian charity of over 200 million dollars! (Canadian Cancer Society, 2010).

Corporate sponsors listed on The Canadian Cancer Society's 2009/2010 Annual Report include corporate giants, Abbott Laboratories, Pfizer Canada Inc., Sanofi-Aventis Canada Inc., Merck-Frosst Canada Ltd., Novartis Pharmaceuticals Canada Inc. and Wyeth Canada (Canadian Cancer Society, 2010).

Why would pharmaceutical companies sponsor charities raising money for cancer?

Do you think it is so the charities will continue to funnel their massive cash flows directly to pharmaceutical research?

Incidentally, *Reuters Health Information* reported in April 2010: US Prescription Drug Sales Hit $300 Billion in 2009, and that's only the United States! (Reuters Health Information, 2010).

Many people believe the cancer industry is *still* trying to find a cure, but we can hear the deception in their messages ringing clear as the grandest bell of all.

The truth is, *we already **have** natural cures for cancer*! We just have to stop believing the hype about them and get to **know** them ourselves!

You know when you *know* something, but do you really **know** it? Really **know** that natural cures for cancer have worked for thousands, maybe millions of people already, and really **know** that conventional treatments like chemotherapy and radiation very rarely work to save peoples' lives, if at all.

People who really **know,** cure cancer using natural therapies **only** and have done so throughout time. Now that we really **know**, we will no longer be able to allow millions of innocent people to be pushed through the *cancer mill*. Truth brings responsibility . . .

How many millions have already been lost to toxic, experimental chemicals like chemotherapy?

When will enough of our loved ones die before we **embrace** the truth and make the necessary changes in our world?

It is blatantly obvious that the cancer industry will never find a cure. They are willing to take money from misled people who have lost their loved ones and give it solely to studies promoting chemotherapy and other toxic treatments.

In February of 2009, The Canadian Cancer Society and the National Cancer Institute of Canada merged to become the Canadian Cancer Society Research Institute. They state, "The Canadian Cancer Society Research Institute is the new research granting function with the

Canadian Cancer Society." (Canadian Cancer Society Research Institute, 2010).

I have a question for the Canadian Cancer Society Research Institute, responsible for distributing the hundreds of millions of dollars collected annually:

When **will** you stop **looking** for a cure and acknowledge *we already have it*?

The Terry Fox Foundation, The Canadian Breast Cancer Foundation and the Breast Cancer Society send the money they collect to the Canadian Cancer Society Research Institute. Even though they collect millions of dollars for cancer research every single year, year after year, very little if any of this money is allocated to herbal and alternative therapies.

How is it that this money is not going towards research in herbal and alternative therapies, when people are walking around alive and well and cancer-free, because they used those therapies?

Salary disclosure figures for executive positions are not available, so we can only guess at how much executives are raking in. Apparently nonprofit organizations are not required to disclose the salaries of their executives in Canada. Why is the Canadian government protecting nonprofit executives by not requiring them to disclose their salaries? It is partly our money given as donations for the love of suffering and dead members of our families and communities that pay these salaries. Why don't we know how much they are?

In Canada, physician income is tied to quantity of patient visits, procedures performed, tests ordered and drugs prescribed, but too often than not, physicians seem far removed from the drugs and tests they order for their patients.

In some cases, physicians prescribe harmful drugs that cause permanent damage to the body's organs, drugs that have not been sufficiently tested, drugs that are improperly used or drugs that are taken in deadly combinations with other drugs.

Patients are advised to stop eating foods that naturally thin their blood and instead take prescribed, dangerous and expensive drugs that are designed to do the same thing, sometimes coming with a huge list of troubling side effects and adverse reactions, some even deadly.

Some physicians order tests upon tests, with no regard for the amount of patient exposure to poisonous dyes or radioactive isotopes.

Some remove vital organs like gall bladders, all the while *pooh-poohing* the fact that simple, inexpensive cleanses remove the stones and blockages, and leave the vital gall bladder in place, improving almost every function of the body!

Nutritional deficiencies are often ignored and many patients never get simple tests that show exactly which vitamins or minerals are at low, unhealthy levels. Fundamental rules of nutrition are never taught to physicians, hence they are never relayed to their patients.

Complementary therapies are embraced because they can be used *alongside* chemotherapy and radiation, and are being heavily marketed with conventional treatments, suggesting that cancer treatment centers are interested in natural treatments. Don't be fooled. The real alternative therapies are abhorred, always being sloughed off like they are unimportant and ineffective. Why? Because they *replace* conventional treatments. How many times have we been told not to rely on natural therapies because they have not been proven by double blind placebo controlled studies?

It all sounds like a really bad horror movie. The profit driven focus of the medical industry takes caring intelligent physicians and turns them into money seeking robots. It kind of reminds me of the 1970s movie, *The Stepford Wives.*

Our present system ironically uses the caring professions to promote the abuse of our families and friends at any cost. We are paying huge financial, spiritual and emotional costs, and the physical costs; we are literally paying with our lives.

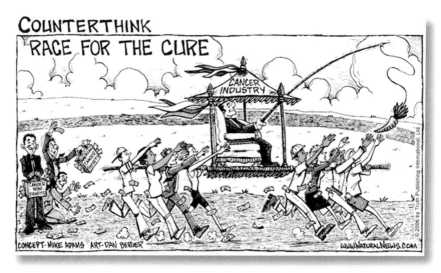

Reprint Courtesy: Cartoon created by Mike Adams of www.NaturalNews.com.

8   You Don't Have To Die

It is the spring of 2004. I find Hoxsey's original 1957 text, *You Don't Have To Die, The Amazing Story of the Hoxsey Cancer Treatment* on eBay. I buy the text from an antique book dealer, then wait impatiently for it to arrive. The photos of patients before and after treatments with Hoxsey's formulas are shocking and amazing!

Harry talks about Mandus Johnson of Galesburg, Illinois. When Harry met Mandus on March 2 of 1930, he had a large cancer that was covering the top of his head. The tumor had consumed Mandus's scalp, his skull was exposed, and more than a pint of 'pus' was drained from beneath the tumor every day. Harry claimed it was the worst case of cancer he had ever seen (Hoxsey, 1957).

Medical officials lied in a public announcement when they said Hoxsey had killed Mandus Johnson. Outraged, supporters of Hoxsey gathered to let the world know that Mandus Johnson was alive and well (Hoxsey, 1957).

The caption on the photo of Mandus in *You Don't Have To Die* reads, "32,000 people turned out in a demonstration in Muscatine, Iowa on May 30, 1930, to witness the 'resurrection' of Mandus Johnson. Cancer covered the top of his skull. Fully healed, he lived on for 20 years."

One photo shows a woman with a huge rotting cancer on her breast, bigger than my fist; the next shows the breast completely healed, with only a scar left to show where the massive tumor once lived. The caption reads, "Mrs. Ethel Dennis of Philadelphia, treated for cancer of the breast in 1934. Before and after treatment. Biopsy report from well-known laboratory, attests that this patient had cancer when our treatment began" (Hoxsey, 1957).

The back cover of Harry's 1957 book states that he was 54 years old at the time of writing. Harry was, "kicked, hounded, persecuted and prosecuted for 35 of those years because he treated cancer with his own herbal medicines, instead of surgery, x-rays and radiation treatments" (Hoxsey, 1957).

Many of these herbs have been used for centuries by Native American healers to treat cancer. They all have cleansing and supportive qualities but, most important, anti-cancer and anti-fungal compounds. The work of eminent botanist, James Duke, Ph.D, formerly of the United States Department of Agriculture shows that all the *Hoxsey* herbs have known anti-cancer, cleansing and detoxifying properties (Dr. Duke's *Phytochemical and Ethnobotanical Databases*, 1998).

The herbs in Hoxsey's formula are also cited in *Plants Used Against Cancer A Survey*, a global summary of folk usage of medicinal plants compiled by chemist Jonathan Hartwell, while at the National Cancer Institute. The compendium was last published in 1984 (Hartwell, 1984).

Harry Hoxsey describes his basic oral medicine, it's benefits and ingredients. The medicine stimulates the body to eliminate toxins, correcting blood chemistry and normalizing cell metabolism. Harry always used Potassium Iodide, mixed with some or all of the following herbs, depending on the situation: Licorice root, Red Clover flowers, Burdock root, Stillingia root, Berberis root, Poke root, Cascara Sagrada, Prickly Ash bark and Buckthorn bark (Hoxsey, 1957).

Everyone should know the war on cancer is largely a fraud.

Dr. Linus Pauling, Two-time Nobel Prize Winner.

9 Experimenting With Herbal Medicine

In the late spring of 2004, I begin experimenting with Harry Hoxsey's formula. The herbs are all listed in his original 1957 text, *You Don't Have To Die*. It is not difficult to make anti-cancer medicine. It's just like preparing any other complex recipe. Herbal teas or tisanes are generally made the same way. Brew a tea with flowers and leaves, and simmer roots, bark and stems on low heat to extract the properties, then combine the teas. Simple.

Most of the herbs are easy to find. Some grow in my garden and wild in the fields around my home. Some are stocked by our local Master Herbalist. I have plenty of opportunities to test my formula over the next few years.

A lump appears on my friends nose. It is not a pimple, is not going away, and is slowly increasing in size. Months go by and it is still there. She feels it is a small basal cell carcinoma. I believe her because she has seen many cancers. She is a nurse.

QUERY HERBS IN THE FORMULA

It is interesting to query the herbs in this formula. Red Clover has literally thousands of chemicals present, hundreds displaying anti-cancer, anti-tumor and anti-fungal properties. To search yourself query James Duke's, *Phytochemical and Ethnobotanical Database*, U.S. Department of Agriculture go to:
http://www.ars-grin.gov/duke/

Do a Plant Search
- Choose *Chemicals and Activities in a particular plant*
- **Enter the name of the plant**
- **Submit query**
- If there is more than one plant, choose the first one with the proper name
- **Click the radio button** *Print Activities with Chemicals*
- **Submit query**
- **Scroll down** until you find the chemicals with anti-cancer properties

We decide to try the tea. She soaks cotton swabs in the tea and keeps them with her. Several times a day she dabs her nose with the tea. Within a couple of weeks the lump is completely gone.

Later that summer we play in a baseball tournament. We spend several hours in the hot sun. The lump returns. Again she dabs the tea on the lump, but this time she applies the medicine consistently until the lump permanently disappears. In May of 2009, Julie's nose has a tiny indent where the lump had been five years ago.

The spot on my nose had been present for about one year. I pre-moistened several q-tips with the tea and stored them in a tiny glass jar. I kept them handy, on my person and regularly applied them to the spot on my nose. It was raised and discolored.

I applied the tea about ten times a day for three weeks, until the lump disappeared. Not long afterward, my nose was exposed all day to the sun during a baseball tournament. The lump returned. Over the next few weeks it resumed its original condition.

I began applying as before, but this time I applied consistently for 3 months.

It is now five years later. The lump has never returned, but there is a tiny scar where it used to be. The scar is almost invisible.

Julie E., Registered Practical Nurse, May 2009.
Julie's name has been changed to protect her identity.

10   CT Scans and Radiation Exposure

It is late 2004. A CT scan shows three tumors in my mother's right lung and one in her bronchial tube. My mother knows there is a tumor in her bronchial tube because it causes her to cough all the time.

CT scans involve much higher doses of radiation than plain-film radiography. This results in a dangerous increase in radiation exposure to anyone having a scan and especially to those having multiple scans. CT scans may find cancer, but they also cause it.

CT scans seem to be a useful diagnostic tool, but they are causing the very disease they are designed to detect. We should not forget that we are irradiating humans and there is something inherently and terribly wrong with this. My mother's body is already dealing with cancer. Why cause more?

In 'Computed Tomography - An Increasing Source of Radiation Exposure,' published in *The New England Journal of Medicine*, the authors show that survivors of the 1945 atomic bombing of Japan with radiation induced cancers, were exposed to similar amounts of radiation as those used in conventional medical diagnostic radioactive scans. The review compiles organ doses from various radiologic studies. Ionizing radiation is measured in mGy (milligrays) or mSv (millisieverts). Dental radiography exposes the brain to 0.005 mGy's. A Posterior-anterior chest radiography exposes the lung to 0.01 mGy's. The danger becomes clear when you consider abdominal CT scan exposes the stomach to 10 mGy's, and a barium enema exposes the colon to 15 mGy's (Brenner, David J., Hall, Eric J., Phil, D., 2007).

The overall risk of cancer was significantly increased in the subgroup of survivors who received radiation at low doses ranging from 5 to 150 mGy's, the mean dose being 40 mGy's, about the amount an adult would receive from two or three CT scans (Brenner, David J., Hall, Eric J., Phil, D., 2007).

The *Radiologyinfo.org* website (a joint effort by the American College of Radiology and the Radiological Society of North America), displays a chart in the article, 'Radiation Exposure in X-ray and CT Examinations,' which shows the radiation dose you are receiving during any procedure. A CT scan of your chest exposes you to 7 mSv or two years equivalent of natural background radiation, an abdominal CT scan exposes you to 10 mSv or three years exposure. According to the article, "to explain in simple terms, we can compare the radiation exposure from one chest x-ray as equivalent to the amount of radiation exposure one experiences from our natural surroundings in 10 days." One chest x-ray has an approximate effective radiation dose of .1 mSv. This means an abdominal CT scan which exposes you to 10 mSv is the equivalent of having 100 chest x-rays! (Radiological Society of North America, 2010).

Most people don't have just one scan at a time. A review of over 33,700 consecutive CT examinations performed in 1998 and 1999, at the Department of Radiology, University of New Mexico Health Sciences Center in Albuquerque, showed patients were having multiple scans (Mettler, Wiest, Locken, Kelsey, 2000).

The review showed during 1990 to 1999, CT examinations increased from 6.1% to 11.1% of all radiology procedures. Of all patients seen in the University of New Mexico's Radiology Department, 19% had at least one CT scan and more than half of them had multiple scans on the same day. Of all patients, 36% had prior CT examination at an earlier time. Children up to age 15 comprised 11.2% of CT scans, but most scans were performed on people aged 36 to 50 years (Mettler, Wiest, Locken, Kelsey, 2000).

In a Yale survey, 'Diagnostic CT Scans: Assessment of Patient, Physician, and Radiologist Awareness of Radiation Dose and Possible Risks,' a shocking 75% of radiologists and emergency-room physicians significantly underestimated the radiation dose from a CT scan. Over half of radiologists, 53% and almost all, an unbelievable 91% of emergency-room physicians did not believe their patient's lifetime risk for cancer was increased with CT scans (Lee, Haims, Monico, Brink, Forman, 2004).

Even more disturbing, only 3% of patients surveyed, believed they were at increased cancer risk after having a CT scan. It is not only physicians who are far removed from the dangers of standard medical tools and treatments. The study concludes that patients are not told about the risks, benefits and radiation dose for CT scans, and that neither patients, emergency department physicians nor radiologists could accurately estimate how much radiation a patient was receiving (Lee, Haims, Monico, Brink, Forman, 2004).

Why don't physicians and radiologists know the cancer risks involved for their patients?

Why don't patients know the risks before they agree to be irradiated?

Recent research reported in 'Radiation from CT scans linked to cancers, deaths,' shows that every year in the United States, 29,000 people may get cancers directly from the past use of CT scans and of those 29,000, about half, 14,500 people, will die from those cancers! (Szabo, 2009).

When I ask my mother how many CT scans she has had, she cannot remember. *"Lots,"* she says.

Months after my mother passes, I find a handwritten record of CT scans and other tests and treatments she endured from March 2003 until May 2004, just over a one year period.

The list of procedures ordered includes, four CT scans (abdominal and chest), one bone scan, two chemotherapy sessions, an MRI on her brain, two heart ultrasounds, hand surgery, bronchoscopy with surgery, and brachytherapy radiation to the bronchi.

In a one year period from CT scans alone, she is exposed to the equivalent radiation of more than 400 chest x-rays.

This does not include the exposure from radiation delivered to her bones through the bone scan, radioactive dye administered during the bone scan or radiation therapy to her bronchi.

MY MOTHER'S ONE YEAR RECORD OF RADIATION AND CHEMOTHERAPY EXPOSURE
(Not including surgeries)

March 13/03	CT Scan
Sept 2/03	CT Scan
Sept 2/03	Bone Scan with radioactive dye
Jan 10/04	CT Scan
Mar 12/04	Brachytherapy radiation in bronchi
Apr 5/04	CT Scan
May 3/04	Chemotherapy
May 17/04	Chemotherapy

After huge amounts of exposure to radiation, doctors inject her with toxic chemotherapy.

A healthy thirty-year old would have a difficult time dealing with this tortuous treatment, let alone my seventy-one year old mother, with all she had been through already . . .

Throughout the 1980s, the National Cancer Institute's (U.S.) advisory board was chaired by Armand Hammer, the Chief Executive Officer of Occidental Petroleum.

While he served as a senior adviser to the NCI, Hammer's firm produced more than 100 billion tons of toxic chemicals, including those that created the superfund toxic waste site at Love Canal and led to the contamination of lush Mississippi River delta towns in Calcacieu Parish.

Devra Davis, 2007.

11   Tea Expels Dead Tumors

In January of 2005 my mother begins therapy with my herbal anti-cancer tea, Bitter Tonic Tea. Within days she starts to look and feel better, her energy increases and she seems much happier.

In May of 2005, after taking the tea for a couple months she begins to have bouts of coughing for two or three days at a time. At least three of them culminate in her coughing out a small round pea like thing, along with a bit of blood and mucous. Then the coughing stops for several weeks until she begins another bout. We believe the hunks of tissue are small solid tumors.

We take a larger, coughed up tumor into her Thoracic Surgeon's office. My mother asks his nurse if this is a normal occurrence and she replies, "No, I have never heard of anyone coughing up tumors before."

I ask Julie E. for her opinion, my friend and nurse who works in palliative care, often with late stage cancer patients. "Even lung cancer patients don't cough up tumors. They cough up blood and mucous though," she says.

Interesting . . .

Tumors don't just let go and come out unless they are dead. They grow and multiply in a never ending proliferation feeding on the body they inhabit. They are attached by blood vessels, which is evident in the tumor we examine. It has a large hole in the middle, is round like a chick pea, and is surrounded by a layer of white tissue. It looks almost fatty. Could it be a layer of immune cells that forms the white layer on the outside of the tumor, I wonder? Natural Killer Cells are immune cells that attack and destroy cancer cells. They are large white cells.

Imagine your body killing cancer. A killer cell migrates toward a cancer cell, then moves close over its plasma membrane. Death Ligands (proteins) from the killer cell connect with Death Receptors on the cell's membrane then pass through. Once inside, it causes a series of events to proceed, which results in the cell digesting itself. Once the cytoskeleton contents and walls of the cell have been fully broken down, macrophages move in to eat up and take away the remains. This process is called apoptosis. Although this process takes place inside a cancerous cell, it is triggered by natural killer cells from your immune system (Berry, 2006).

To see this process in action watch the video by Drew Berry, 'Apoptosis and Signal Transduction,' at http://www.wehi.edu.au/education/wehitv/apoptosis_and_signal_transduction/

Histopathology Report

In late May we receive a pathology report which shows the one centimeter tumor is consistent with metastasized bowel cancer. This means my mother coughed up a bowel tumor that had spread to her lung. Below is a photo of the lab report after the larger tumor was analyzed.

You can see my mother's handwriting. She doesn't agree with the report that the tumor is a fragment, as we both know it's a whole tumor. She writes, "I don't believe! Not a fragment!"

Notice the report states, "No non-tumorous tissue identified." This is true, the dead tumor is the only thing that came out. There was no lung tissue expelled, only tumor!

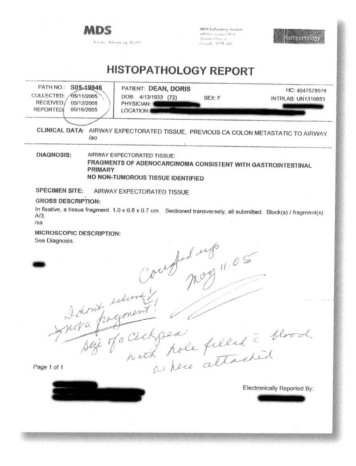

The surgeon tells my mother, "Keep doing what you are doing," but never once, does he ask for information about what caused the tumor to come out.

In June of 2005, another CT scan shows no further metastases in her lung, no further tumor growth in her bronchial tube or trachea. After six months of taking the anti-cancer tea she has gained twenty pounds. She looks amazing and feels great. She is quilting, visiting friends and family, and *bombing* around in her little car. She definitely does not appear to be *dying of cancer*.

Unfortunately, after several months she stops taking the tea. She complains that it is too strong and irritating on what is left of her stomach and re-sectioned bowel.

She has constant digestive and bowel problems from two stomach surgeries. The 1970s seemed to be a boom for stomach *ulcer* surgeries, as there were four in my family alone: my father had two surgeries and my mother had two as well.

By the end of the 1970s, Herberman's lab at the National Cancer Institute showed that natural killers (cells) are on high alert for cells that are in the wrong place at the wrong time. They can immediately identify potentially metastatic cells that have broken out of their original location and entered the blood, and quickly eliminate most if not all of them.

Devra Davis, 2007.

12   Is Cancer A Fungus?

Dr. Tullio Simoncini is an Italian doctor, specializing in oncology (cancer), diabetology and metabolic disorders. He also thinks the white tissue surrounding the tumor is made up of Natural Killer Cells. He believes the growth of a fungal colony, together with the reaction of the tissue trying to defend itself and the presence of immune cells, all cause the tumor or mass to form.

Coincidentally, or not . . . the medical dictionary places *candida* directly after *cancer* . . .

From the 'Cancer is a Fungus' website:

A fungal infection always forms the basis of every neoplastic formation (formation of new tissue as in a cancerous tumor), and this formation tries to spread within the whole organism without stopping.

Dr. Tullio Simoncini, 2010.

Normally our immune system kills fungal cells wherever they are found, but when our body is polluted and fungi are being fed sugar continuously, colonies of yeast begin to form, mature and spread and can get out of control as the immune system struggles to keep up.

Dr. Simoncini uses the simplest of therapies, $NaHCO_3$ or sodium bicarbonate, to *miraculously* cure many different forms of cancer. He uses a variety of methods to get the sodium bicarbonate into the mass. He applies the sodium bicarbonate topically, injects it into or near the tumorous site, or uses oral therapy.

In 'Bicarbonate Increases Tumor pH and Inhibits Spontaneous Metastases,' the authors state, acid pH has been shown to stimulate tumor cell invasion and metastasis. Sodium Bicarbonate or $NaHCO_3$ increased the pH in tumors enough to inhibit spreading. Oral $NaHCO_3$ selectively increased the pH of tumors and reduced the formation of spontaneous metastases in mouse models of metastatic breast cancer, and splenic injection 'significantly' reduced hepatic (liver cell) metastases. After injecting the $NaHCO_3$ into the mice's tails, the results showed that it inhibited prostate cancer cells (Robey, Bagget, Kirkpatrick, Roe, Dosescu, Sloane, et al., 2009).

Watch the closing chapter of *Cancer - The Forbidden Cures*, at http://thegoodwitch.ca/cancer-is-a-fungus/ (the video takes a minute to load) as Simoncini discusses his 'Cancer is a Fungus' theory and his simple cure. He shows many photos of internal cancers and points out how these tumors are made up of colonies of the common fungus, Candida Albicans; together with our tissues' and immune system's reactions.

Need more? Check out Dr. Simoncini's remarkable therapy at his website, CancerIsAFungus.com.

The Land and Seed Theory

Traditional Ayurveda, describes the theory of immunity, the *beej-bhumi*, or 'Land and Seed' theory, as a metaphor for how cancer is able to take hold in our body. This Ayurvedic philosophy is synonymous with the theory that *cancer is a fungus*.

Our body is the land, and cancer is the seed. In this case, we do not want our bodies to be fertile. If the environment inside our body *is fertile*, or toxic, sweet and acidic, cancer feeds off our tissues and organs, weakening them. When it's growth and reproduction is supported . . . it takes hold and flourishes.

When our body is *infertile*, or alkaline, clean, and oxygenated, with no excess sugar or congestion, which does not support the growth of cancer, it is not able to colonize and disrupt our living system. Our immune system kills and discards it.

Cancer = Fungus

Aflatoxins found in moldy peanuts and grains are known to be one of the strongest carcinogenic substances to humans and animals. This means we have known for a long time that fungi cause cancer, because aflatoxins are toxins from fungi! Aflatoxins are commonly found on moldy grains, peanuts and legumes. Always buy these goods fresh and keep them refrigerated. If they smell or taste off in the slightest manner, discard them immediately.

Aflatoxin: 'A toxin produced by some strains of *Aspergillus flavus* and *A. parasiticus* that causes cancer in laboratory animals. It may be present in peanuts and other seeds contaminated with *Aspergillus* molds. It is not practical to try to remove alflatoxin from contaminated foods in order to make them edible' (Venes & Thomas, 2001).

Alflatoxicosis: 'Poisoning caused by ingestion of peanuts or peanut products contaminated with *Aspergillus flavus* or other *Aspergillus* strains that produce aflatoxin. Farm animals and humans are susceptible to this toxicosis' (Venes & Thomas, 2001).

FUNGAL CELLS	CANCER CELLS
Spread by chlamydospores, cells that flake off, float through the bloodstream and settle in other places	Spread by cells that break off from the original tumor, float through the bloodstream and settle in other places. Does it really matter what they are called?
Live in an anaerobic environment with little or no oxygen	Live in an anaerobic environment with little or no oxygen
Live in an acid environment because alkalinity kills them	Live in an acid environment because alkalinity kills them
Sugar makes them grow wild and crazy	Sugar makes them grow wild and crazy
Garlic kills them	Garlic kills them
Sodium bicarbonate kills them	Sodium bicarbonate kills them
Herbs that kill candida with anti-fungal properties also kill cancer with anti-cancer properties	Herbs that kill cancer cells with anti-cancer properties also kill candida fungi with anti-fungal properties

If you need more proof that cancer is caused by a fungus, consider a study by X. Hong, Y. Chou and J. Lazareff, published in *Surgical Neurology* in July of 2008.

You can see the abstract at *Surgical Neurology*, 'Brain stem candidiasis mimicking cerebellopontine angle tumor.' Here: http://www.surgicalneurology-online.com/article/S0090-3019%2808%2900009-8/abstract

The study shows that infection by Candida Albicans in the brain of a seventeen month old boy was thought to be a cerebral tumor.

The boy underwent right retrosigmoid craniotomy and excisional biopsy, to determine that he was really infected with fungus!

The boy recovered completely after a year long antifungal treatment. At two year followup the boy was 'well, without neurological problems' (Hong, Chou and Lazareff, 2008).

In 'Electron microscopy reveals fungal cells within tumor tissue from two African patients with AIDS-associated Kaposi sarcoma,' a biopsy from two African patients revealed fungal cells of Candida Albicans within the tumor tissue, even though the patients showed no signs of a systemic fungal infection (Marquart, 2006).

David Holland, M.D. of *ThinkFungus.com* wrote an interesting story about a nurse at http://www.loveoffering.com/fungus.htm

The nurse worked in a bone marrow transplant center. The nurse became sick and was diagnosed with leukemia. Doctors treated her with chemotherapy, which *apparently* caused a secondary fungal infection, which she was then treated for with antifungal drugs. The leukemia went into remission. Later it returned and doctors again wanted her to go through grueling chemotherapy treatments, the thought of which caused her to seek out a second opinion, and this time the pathologist told the nurse she didn't have leukemia, but a fungal infection! She was treated for the fungal infection and to this day is fine (Holland, 2010).

YEAST INFECTIONS

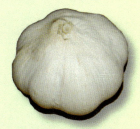

Garlic – the wonder cure – it is antifungal, antibacterial, antiviral, anti-worm, antiparasitic.

Our family uses raw fresh garlic to quickly eradicate yeast infections. Withdrawing their food supply by not eating sugar helps too! We have used this method in my own home for years, when sugar consumption or antibiotic use has caused yeast infections in my children. Now we take fresh garlic instead of antibiotics for all infections!

This method has been used for centuries, long before modern medicine invented chemically based antifungals. For topical yeast infections, crush a clove of garlic in warm water and apply often with a soft compress. External yeast infections clear within hours using this method. To read more about using garlic to clear infections, go to '*Garlic Remedy*' at **http://thegoodwitch.ca/garlic-remedy/**

This situation raises some serious questions. What if leukemia is ALWAYS caused by a fungal infection? What if all the children with leukemia (and adults), being treated with toxic chemotherapy, really need natural antifungals and a change in diet? This would mean that leukemia patients are being needlessly hurt and in many cases, killed!

Back to sodium bicarbonate for a minute. What is it about sodium bicarbonate and why does it kill fungi or cancer cells so readily?

Dr. Tullio Simoncini, the Italian oncologist, claims complete cures of breast and other cancers within days using only sodium bicarbonate – nothing else!

Sodium bicarbonate ($NaHCO_3$): a white odorless powder with saline taste . . . used to treat acidosis (e.g. in renal failure). Orally it is used as an antacid . . . externally it is used as a mild alkaline wash (Venes & Thomas, 2001).

The alkaline nature of baking soda, with a pH of slightly over 8, is enough to allow more oxygen into the cell walls, killing the acid loving, oxygen hating, anaerobic Candida Albicans. Sodium bicarbonate is alkaline which makes it a powerful fungal killer. Cancer cells or fungal cells, whatever we call them, **cannot grow** in an alkaline environment! Baking soda is a cheap and effective therapy for killing cancer!

When I was a child we regularly mixed a teaspoon of baking soda with fresh lemon juice and water. My parents taught us this remedy which instantly cured acid in our stomachs. It is too bad they did not know what else sodium bicarbonate was capable of . . .

DAMP FUNGI ON SEEDLINGS

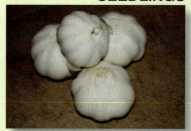

Growing vegetable seedlings for my garden taught me the benefits of using garlic to kill fungi. During a spring with low light and cool weather, my tomato seedlings get *Damp*, a fungi that causes them to shrivel from the root all the way up the stem. Once *Damp* gets hold, you can see it spread across the tray in a trail of devastation over the baby plants, killing all of them within a couple of days.

You can use the same method for killing Damp fungus on seedlings as used to kill yeast infections. One or two applications of fresh garlic water will kill all fungus and any baby plants not yet affected by the fungus, will be sitting straight up and healthy the next day. It really works!

Baking soda can play a part in re-alkalizing your body, it's fluids and tissues, but it is important to remember that eating properly will do this naturally. Making the blood alkaline by eating more fresh, natural, mineral rich foods and reducing acidic foods, not only kills cancer, but improves functioning of all parts of your body. It will ensure that no other fungal colonies will ever be able to live in your body again! More about this later, in the 10 Key Healing Principles . . .

In the article, 'Will ARM & HAMMER Baking Soda work as an antacid?' authors suggest taking half a teaspoon of baking soda in four ounces of water (about half a glass) every two hours, or as directed by a physician. They warn to not take more than seven half teaspoons, or three half teaspoons if you are over sixty years old, in twenty-four hours, and to not use the maximum dosage for more than two weeks. Baking soda is high in sodium, over 1200 mg per teaspoon and can have contraindications with medications and medical conditions like high blood pressure and liver disease. Never administer baking soda to a child under five years of age. Also, never take baking soda in its powder form as its alkalinity can cause serious damage if not mixed with water first. Consult with a qualified practitioner before taking baking soda as a therapeutic agent (Church & Dwight Co., Inc., 2008).

My family uses one teaspoon of baking soda in a full glass of water daily, for a couple of days while eating mineral rich greens and avoiding acid causing sugar, meat, dairy and grains, to rebalance our pH levels; while testing on a pH urine strip. See 'How to test my own pH' at http://thegoodwitch.ca/how-to-test-my-own-ph/.

Symptoms of chronic Candida infection

What are the symptoms of a chronic Candida infection? The symptoms of Candida infection vary so widely, it is often difficult to determine which symptoms are actually related to Candida, which means infections are often left undiagnosed.

Mild symptoms can include: cold sweats, cravings for sugar (bread, alcohol, pastries, cake, potato chips, grains, fruits, dried fruits, ice cream, candies, pasta, cheese or anything dairy), cravings for salt, coated tongue, intestinal gas, indigestion, acne, vaginal, anal, skin or scalp itching, nail ridges, brown 'liver' spots, muscle twitching, weight gain and feeling jumpy.

Serious symptoms include: depression, insomnia, weakness, slow pulse, hives, fatigue, excessive hair loss, heart palpitations, kidney problems, difficulty urinating, eczema, psoriasis, weight loss, diarrhea, nightmares, pounding headaches and cancer (1986, Trowbridge & Walker).

Finally Candida can manifest in horrific symptoms. After my father's final dose of toxic chemotherapy, his immune cells died off and Candida was free to completely take over his body. We could see the white foaming mass of fungi growing up his throat, into and throughout his mouth and nose. The infection made his throat so raw, it was impossible for him to swallow food. This is known as systemic Candidiasis, worst on the scale of Candida infections.

The above symptoms are far from a full list of the hundreds of symptoms related to infection by Candida Albicans.

13 More Radiation Exposure

It is the spring of 2005 and my girlfriend Nancy, is diagnosed with breast cancer. She has surgery and radiation. Doctors tell her they are concerned the cancer may have spread to her bones. She begins regular screening for bone cancer through radioactive bone scans.

It does not take long before she is diagnosed with metastasized breast cancer in her bones. Could it have been the radioactive bone scans?

Nancy is also being treated with Tamoxifen. When I look up Tamoxifen, I find out that it is itself a carcinogen or cancer causing substance.

I give Nancy the recipe for tea. She starts taking it. After a few months she tells me, doctors say her disease is still progressing, but more slowly than before. It must be the chemotherapy they tell her.

She does well on the tea for about six months. I visit her periodically. We sit on her porch, drinking tea and discussing her cancer situation. She is in good spirits and seems well, but over several months I can tell the radiation and chemotherapy treatments are taking their toll on her. Her back seems hunched over and I fear cancer is spreading inside her bones.

I lose contact with her for about nine months and wonder why she has not called. Her sister calls me. Nancy has died a painful death from bone cancer.

I am extremely angry. Why did she trust them? I rack my brains trying to make sense of her death. The strange thing is this: Two of my girlfriends were diagnosed with breast cancer only weeks apart.

Nancy's tumor is not invasive doctors tell her. It is encapsulated, growing ever larger, not invading surrounding tissues. It is the *safe* kind of breast cancer. She has a lumpectomy and radiation. She later dies from bone cancer, metastasized from primary cancer of the breast.

My other friend, Marilou, who is diagnosed with invasive breast cancer, the *dangerous* one, has the same treatments, lumpectomy and radiation. She is still alive in 2010, with no recurrence.

The difference? Nancy has bone scans, as her physician wants to *make sure* the cancer is not in her bones. Marilou's physician sees no need for bone scans. Could this be the reason Marilou is still alive?

Is it possible that bone scans caused Nancy's bone cancer? Is it possible that injecting radioactive dye inside someone's bones repeatedly, or even once, can cause bone cancer to occur?

The Technician at the Radiology Department of my local hospital explains the protection provided for the syringe carrying the radioactive material that is injected into a person, before the bone scan is performed:

We use a metal container carrying lead shields. Inside the lead shields are syringes filled with methylene diphosphanate, tagged to the radioisotope, Technetium 99 known as TC99M.

Radiology Technician, 2009.

I ask him how he is protected against absorbing the radiation. He says,

I am exposed because I stand right beside the patient, so the amount I get is monitored regularly.

Radiology Technician, 2009.

But . . . is *monitoring* the doses of radiation you are receiving *really* the same as *protection*?

This radioactive diagnostic tool is used to detect cancer in the bones of women who already have breast cancer. I *believe* it causes cancer to occur in the bones of people being scanned, whether or not they have breast cancer.

For six months I search for information about bone scans. I finally find what I am looking for. Radiation *accumulates* in the skeletal system. MDS Nordion S.A. Belgium's, 'Kit for Preparation of Technetium Medronate Injection,' download at http://www.health.gov.il/units/pharmacy/trufot/alonim/822.pdf

The report states, Technetium-99m *accumulates* in the skeletal system, up to 36% in healthy people and by as much as 45% in people with cancer that has already spread. They tell us, "Any exposure to ionizing radiation is linked with cancer induction" (notice they said *any exposure*). Lastly, they say, "There have been no safety studies," on the cancer causing ability of their Technetium-99m injection.

What, no safety studies? Why not?

MDS Nordion Canada's 'Fact Sheets' for radioisotope products state, 'verification of their suitability for use in humans is the sole responsibility of the purchaser' (MDS Inc. 1, 2008).

Why would it say that?

Is it possible they are *not* suitable for use in humans?

Why wouldn't their suitability for use in humans already be established?

According to MDS Nordion's 'Annual Information Form' for 2007, "approximately 18 million scans are performed each year and 80% use a Tc99m radiopharmaceutical" (MDS Inc. 2, 2008).

I look upon cancer in the same way that I look upon heart disease, arthritis, high blood pressure, or even obesity, for that matter, in that by dramatically strengthening the body's immune system through diet, nutritional supplements, and exercise, the body can rid itself of the cancer, just as it does in other degenerative diseases. Consequently, I wouldn't have chemotherapy and radiation because I'm not interested in therapies that cripple the immune system, and, in my opinion, virtually ensure failure for the majority of cancer patients.

Dr Julian Whitaker, M.D.

14 Rene Caisse and Essiac™

It is the fall of 2005. I am teaching an alternative health course at a local college. A student does a presentation on Essiac tea. Her presentation is excellent and gets right to the point. Rene Caisse used her formula to heal thousands of patients, for over fifty years!

Essiac™ is named after Rene Caisse (pronounced Case), a Canadian nurse who claims to have learned her formula from an elderly native woman who used it to recover from breast cancer many years before.

The original formula is sold by various suppliers under different names. None of them is allowed to say what the tea is really used for, but thankfully it's use is widely understood. Most health food stores carry at least one variation of Rene Caisse's formula.

Rene used her first version of the formula on her aunt in 1924, who was diagnosed with inoperable stomach cancer with liver complications. Within one year Rene's aunt was completely healed without reoccurrence (Snow, 1996).

Rene fought for recognition of her formula with the conventional cancer community for over fifty years, but instead of recognition, she was under constant threat of imprisonment.

> ## IT IS SIMPLE TO MAKE YOUR OWN *Native Herbal Cancer Tea* JUST LIKE RENE CAISSE DID . . .
>
> Mix the herbs and keep in a large glass jar in a dark, cool place.
>
> **4 cups Burdock Root**
> **3 1/2 cups Sheep Sorrel**
> **1/2 cup Slippery Elm Bark**
> **1/4 cup Turkish Rhubarb Root**
>
> Place several glass jars, lids and seals in cold water to cover, in a large pot. Bring to boil and boil hard for 10 minutes.
>
> In the meantime, to make the tea, mix one cup of herbal blend to five cups of fresh water. Heat pot of water to boiling. Add the herbs and simmer for five minutes, remove from heat and tighten lid on pot. Let the tea steep for 20 to 30 minutes. Strain the tea through cheesecloth into another pot.
>
> Reheat the tea to boiling and pour into sterilized jars, top with seal and tighten lid. Leave on counter to cool before putting away in refrigerator.
>
> Once a jar is opened, the tea must be used within 30 days, and always kept refrigerated (Adapted from, *The Essence of Essiac,* Snow, 1996).

In 1977, Rene Caisse passed her formula to Resperin Canada Limited, who still sell her formula today, saying it is the only *true* Essiac™ formula. They claim, "'The quality of the ingredients as well as the ratio of the herbs is obviously of prime importance in how the product functions' (Snow, 1996).

I believe their formula is an excellent combination of anti-cancer herbs, just like many others.

Even Rene Caisse did not invent her own formula, she learned it from someone else. The truth is that these formulas belong to no one, and by the end of this book you will have already learned how to make several of your own amazing anti-cancer herbal teas, that may be even more effective than the original Essiac™ formula.

Many people have taken time to study the properties of various herbs and have developed recipes using many combinations of different herbs. Anti-cancer properties can be found in thousands of different plants, which means there are many combinations of herbs that are successful at healing cancer. Anywhere in the world, you will find simple plants, all around you, with secret, potent anti-cancer properties.

Methods of extracting the properties of herbs have been known by natural practitioners for eons. This knowledge is not secret, which means you *can* easily make your own herbal medicines at home.

Last week a woman left a message on my phone asking if I could sell her the *real* Essiac, and I was disappointed to find that her message had been deleted and I had no way to call her back. I wanted to tell her that I do not sell tea, but rather, teach people how to heal themselves. In this way people remain in control and responsible for their own health.
I think it is also important for people to learn to make their own remedies and herbal medicines, use them properly, and be aware of their dangers and interactions with medications, supplements and preexisting conditions like pregnancy and high blood pressure. It is important to *befriend* the herbs you use and know them well.

I also wanted to tell her that it does not matter whether the tea you are using is a variation of Rene Caisse's formula, or the exact formula that Harry Hoxsey's great-grandfather used.

There are a plethora of formulas for anti-cancer herbal medicines, and there are *local* herbs growing in every corner of the earth that kill cancer cells and whole tumors. Many of the herbs used in effective anti-cancer formulas, like Caisse's and Hoxsey's blends, are native to the areas where they lived.

Focusing on finding one *true* formula that cures cancer is fruitless. Any formula that uses known anti-cancer herbs has the potential to kill

45

cancer. Just as a North American anti-cancer formula using red clover works to kill cancer and heal your body, so does a Peruvian blend made with Pau D'Arco, or a Chinese blend made with Ta Huang. It does not matter where you live, the medicinal herbs that grow naturally in your area will work to heal your body.

Buying quality herbs today is not a problem. You can source herbs in bulk from a Master Herbalist or health food store. Better yet, grow the herbs yourself or harvest them from the wild, as did the elderly native woman who taught Rene Caisse how to make anti-cancer herbal tea so many years ago.

If you are harvesting wild herbs it is important to follow safe practices by knowing what you are harvesting and taking only what you need, always leaving behind some plants so they may continue to propagate.

Recently a friend and neighbour of mine wanted to dig up horseradish root from my garden to make horseradish sauce. I showed him the horseradish plant in early summer so he would know which plant to dig up in the fall, the normal time to dig roots.

In early October he came with a garden fork and began digging up the horseradish plant. After he had removed about half of the large plant, I looked out and realized that he was in the wrong spot in my yard. He had actually dug up part of a large Comfrey plant. The plants have similar leaves and an unpracticed eye could easily make this mistake. I am almost positive he would have realized the difference in the smell of the root, but if he had made horseradish sauce from Comfrey roots he could have easily poisoned himself! Comfrey is not a plant to be ingested, but is used topically to relieve pain and heal bruises, sprains, torn ligaments and broken bones.

I must remember to warn friends about the Stinging Nettle patch!

15 Tea Annihilates Suspicious Mole

In the fall of 2005, my friend Donna notices a 'J' shaped mole on her upper thigh. She visits to her physician who says it looks suspicious. She is instructed to watch the mole carefully and to come back if it changes shape.

Several months later the mole begins to fill out. It has jagged edges, has become raised and is even darker in the centre. She shows it to me and we wonder if the tea would help. We figure there is no harm in trying. She soaks a bandaid in the tea and tapes it to her leg. She repeats this procedure nightly. Within days, the mole begins to dry up and peel off in layers.

Three weeks later I am walking around campus between classes with my friend and coworker, Sally. Donna comes flying up in her little car and screeches to a halt when she sees us. She jumps out of the car, lifts the edge of her skirt and says with a smile, "Look . . . No mole!"

We can't believe it. After only two weeks, the mole is completely gone.

A few years ago I noticed that a mole on my upper left thigh which was normally round, had begun to change shape . . . it was no longer round and symmetrical.

It began to take on the shape of the letter J and the center of it began to get darker and darker. I pointed it out to my doctor months later at an annual physical exam. She said, "We'll keep an eye on that."

After a year, the mole began to change again. This time, it became raised and hard and the center was even darker than before. I decided to use Lisa's anti-cancer tea.

I drank a little of it from time to time but what REALLY worked was applying the tea topically to the mole. I soaked the little gauze part of a Band-Aid and put it over the mole every night for less than 2 weeks and it literally disappeared!

I would recommend that anyone should try using this method on any suspicious moles.

"

Donna G., Registered Nurse, Summer 2008.
Donna's name is changed to protect her identity.

16 Astra Zeneca and Tamoxifen

We have all heard about the conspiracy surrounding cancer treatments and we know that somewhere there must be a cure for cancer, but we do not act like we believe it. Why?

How many times have you thought yourself, or heard someone say, "There is a cure, *they* just don't want us to know."

Why don't *they* want us to know?

I have thought about this for many years and I have come up with some solid answers. Apart from going into exhaustive detail about all the conspiracies surrounding cancer treatment, I would like to give you one excellent example that tells everything.

INTERNATIONAL AGENCY FOR RESEARCH ON CANCER – TAMOXIFEN CITRATE

'Tamoxifen Monograph' at: http://monographs.iarc.fr/ Group 1: Carcinogenic to humans 'Tamoxifen Monograph' – Type Tamoxifen in the search bar. Click on the first entry, CPY document for Tamoxifen to download the complete Monograph in pdf form.

My research exposes the truth about Tamoxifen, the first and most widely used breast cancer treatment, and the drug my friend Nancy was given. Tamoxifen is manufactured by Astra Zeneca, a pharmaceutical giant.

I find the chemical on a list of carcinogens. When I search the database of the International Agency for Research on Cancer, a branch of the World Health Organization, there it is, as plain as the nose on my face:

Tamoxifen, Group 1: Carcinogenic to humans

Tamoxifen has been approved for use as a pharmaceutical since 1970. It's purpose is to block the action of the natural hormone estrogen. Tamoxifen was originally developed as an oral contraceptive, but many studies show that instead of inhibiting ovulation, Tamoxifen stimulates it (IARC, 2010).

There are several other interesting 'Group 1 Carcinogens' listed on the IARC website including:

Estrogen-progestogen menopausal therapy; Estrogen-progestogen oral contraceptives; Estrogens, nonsteroidal; Estrogens, steroidal; Estrogen therapy postmenopausal and Oral contraceptives (IARC, 2010).

It seems that most of these *treatments* are designed to be recommended for women.

When I research further, I find Astra Zeneca is involved in breast cancer in other more haunting ways.

Astra Zeneca is the child of a British company known as ICI, Imperial Chemical Industries. In 1927 the company made a pre-tax profit of 4.5 million british pounds! ICI claims to be the originators of the word "plastic" and are responsible for the plastic technology which has permeated our world, from acrylic windscreens and neon signs to food wrap and plastic squeeze bottles.

ICI began using synthesizing technologies to develop products for the health industry, inventing a treatment for malaria called Paludrine and creating fluothane in 1953, which soon became the most widely used anaesthetic in the western world. By the 1960s, ICI had a product history that included plastics, paints, herbicides, pesticides, explosives, fertilizers, dyestuffs, non-ferrous metals and pharmaceuticals. Julia Kollewe and Graeme Wearden summarize the history of ICI in, 'ICI: from Perspex to Paints' (Kollewe, 2007).

In 'How Chemicals Rose To The Challenge,' Judith Perera reports that Imperial Chemical Industries turned its focus to creating weedkillers from the same chemicals used to manufacture chemicals like Agent Orange, defoliants used to clear large areas of growth which provided cover for insurgent forces during the Vietnam war (Perera, 1985).

In the 1980s ICI reached its peak, becoming the first UK company to reach one billion british pounds in annual pre-tax profits, but it did not last long and by 1993 ICI was in so much trouble that it spun off its pharmaceutical and agrochemical divisions. Astra Zeneca, the pharmaceutical arm, and it's sister company, Zeneca Agrochemicals both emerged from the ashes of Imperial Chemical Industries (Kollewe, 2007).

In a merger with Novartis Agribusiness, Zeneca Agrochemicals changed it's name to Syngenta. Syngenta manufacture selective and non-selective herbicides, fungicides, and insecticides, as well as corn, soybean, flower and vegetable seeds. They *were* one of the world's largest producers of chlorine, and organochlorine pesticides, (some of the world's most dangerous carcinogens, implicated in breast cancer), until in 2004, Syngenta sold off a 75% interest in its sulphur and chlorine based chemicals intermediates business, SF-Chem AG to a private buyer (Securities and Exchange Commission, 2005).

Astra Zeneca manufactures Nolvadex, Istubul, or Valodex (tamoxifen citrate), an oral anti-estrogen widely used in the treatment of breast cancer.

Several studies verify that overexposure of Tamoxifen has the potential to increase the risk of endometrial cancer. Many women treated with Tamoxifen for breast cancer develop uterine cancer, as shown by the large number of reported cases. Many cases of other cancers have been reported after the use of Tamoxifen. Several animal studies reported liver cancers and liver-biliary cancer. Scandinavian studies showed increased risk for gastrointestinal cancers (IARC, 2010).

In several animal studies, hepatocellular carcinomas or liver tumors were found in rats fed higher doses of Tamoxifen. One study involved thirty rats who were fed basal diets or diets with Tamoxifen from six weeks of age. No liver tumors were present in the control rats, but almost all of the treated rats showed at least one liver tumor and some had multiple tumors (Carthew et al., 1995).

Astra Zeneca boasts Nolvadex (Tamoxifen) is the "world's largest selling breast cancer treatment" (Astra Zeneca, 2010).

Nolvadex (Tamoxifen) was approved by the FDA in 1996 for the reduction of breast cancer in women at high risk. Nolvadex has also been approved for reduction of contralateral breast cancer, meaning cancer in the opposite breast of a women who has had cancer in one breast. Astra Zeneca reports that trials are underway for paediatric use of Nolvadex (Astra Zeneca, 2010).

In 2006 Astra Zeneca's Nolvadex was discontinued by Astra Zeneca as generic tamoxifen was widely available, which also means it can be ordered over the internet within twenty-four hours with a prescription.

Now Astra Zeneca is busy trying to prove to physicians and patients that Arimidex, a newer drug under patent, is better than Tamoxifen. Remember that their patent on Tamoxifen has run out! (AstraZeneca United Kingdom, 2010).

Chronic overexposure of Tamoxifen citrate has an accumulative effect and can cause serious or fatal side effects including uterine cancer, strokes and blood clots in the lung (Astra Zeneca Canada Ltd., 2010).

As a chemist trained to interpret data, it is incomprehensible to me that physicians can ignore the clear evidence that chemotherapy does much, much more harm than good.

Alan Nixon, Ph.D., Past President, American Chemical Society.

17 National Breast Cancer Awareness Month and Mammograms

Breast Cancer Awareness Month is the brainchild of Astra Zeneca. A pharmaceutical company that manufactures and sells chemotherapy drugs used in the treatment of breast cancer, created National Breast Cancer Awareness Month . . . to educate us.

According to their website, The National Breast Cancer Awareness Month (NBCAM) partners with government agencies, medical associations and public service organizations.

They all work together to educate us about breast cancer and to share information and provide greater access to breast cancer *screening* services.

Their goals include teaching us to practice regular self-breast exams and making sure we identify any changes since the last time we examined our breasts.

We are encouraged to schedule regular visits with our doctor and have *annual* mammograms, even though *annual* mammograms are discouraged for *all* women by government and medical agencies (NBCAM, 2010).

Health Canada recommends a screening mammogram every two years for women fifty to sixty-nine years of age. Studies have not shown conclusive evidence that regular

---

BREAST CANCER AWARENESS MONTH

Read about Breast Cancer Awareness Month here:
http://www.nbcam.org/about_nbcam.cfm

Notice the copyright in the footnote at the bottom of every page of the website **www.nbcam.org**, National Breast Cancer Awareness Month: It says, "Copyright © 2010, AstraZeneca HealthCare Foundation"

Why do they own the copyright to the NBCAM website?

Does that mean AstraZeneca HealthCare Foundation owns and runs the NBCAM website?

The NBCAM website says that AstraZeneca HealthCare Foundation is the 'principal sponsor' of NBCAM (National Breast Cancer Awareness Month, 2010).

Principal sponsor or owner . . .

What do you think? And . . . does the name really make a difference? It is obvious who is in charge of Breast Cancer Awareness Month.

screening mammograms are beneficial for women under the age of fifty and over the age of sixty-nine. Women outside this range are encouraged to have a diagnostic mammogram, only if recommended by a doctor for a breast lump or other symptom. Women under fifty are *not* encouraged to have regular screening (Health Canada, 2007). Here: http://www.hc-sc.gc.ca/hl-vs/iyh-vsv/med/mammog-eng.php

In December 2009, The U.S. Preventive Services Task Force released its recommendations on breast cancer screening. The report recommends biennial screening mammography for women aged fifty to seventy-four years of age. The Task Force recommends that the decision to start biennial screening in women under the age of fifty remains with the patient, and depends on her values regarding the benefits and harms of biennial screening (U.S. Preventive Services Task Force, 2009) Here: http://www.uspreventiveservicestaskforce.org/uspstf/uspsbrca.htm.

Government guidelines from Canada and the United States do not recommend annual screening mammograms! Only women over fifty are encouraged to have mammograms regularly, but every two years, not annually!

Do you think these guidelines changed because of the mounding evidence showing regular screening by mammograms causes our breasts to accumulate damage from radiation which increases our risk of breast cancer?

NBCAM would like to encourage women to adhere to whatever treatment is prescribed by their doctor, and they stress the importance that women should know *the facts* about recurrence of breast cancer (National Breast Cancer Awareness Month, 2010).

The education we are receiving from National Breast Cancer Awareness Month is biased. It is based on improving the profits of pharmaceutical companies, and includes no information about the causes of cancer, functional nutrition, nutrient deficiencies, toxicity, fungal infections, or improving our immune system's ability to fight cancer . . .

The National Breast Cancer Awareness Month website states that the nonprofit organization, AstraZeneca Healthcare Foundation is the principal sponsor of National Breast Cancer Awareness Month (National Breast Cancer Awareness Month, 2010).

Why is AstraZeneca Healthcare Foundation the principal sponsor and what is the main purpose of National Breast Cancer Awareness Month?

National Breast Cancer Awareness Month teaches *early detection* by promoting annual radioactive mammograms for women. However, studies show that having regular mammograms puts a woman at risk for developing breast cancer. Mammograms do after all, painfully squash your breast between two hard, cold plates, while shooting radioactive x-rays through your compressed breast tissue. According to RadiologyInfo.org, "The effective radiation dose from a mammogram is about 0.7 mSv, which is about the same as the average person receives from background radiation in three months" (Radiological Society of North America, Inc. 2010).

In 'The Canadian National Breast Screening Study-1,' *more* cancers were found in screened women, and the study concluded that mammography, physical examination and self-examination **did not** reduce mortality more than a single exam and instructions on self-examination. The study concludes that screening forty to forty-nine year old women is not likely to reduce breast cancer by twenty percent or more (Miller, To, Baines, Wall, 2002).

Astra Zeneca also coined the well known phrase, 'Early detection is your best protection.' How does finding something after it is there, protect you? Is it possible that early detection gives Astra Zeneca an opportunity to make women with a small, detected breast cancer, a valuable and long term client? Astra Zeneca's total revenue in 2008 was a staggering $31,601,000,000, or more than 31 billion U.S. dollars, but they are not the only pharmaceutical company with such massive revenues (AstraZeneca, 2009).

In 2002, the Fortune 500 listed ten drug companies whose combined *profits (not revenues!)* of $35.9 billion were more than the $33.7 billion in profits for all the other 490 businesses combined, in the Fortune 500 list (Angell, 2004).

In the article, 'Top 17 Paychecks in Big Pharma,' written by Tracy Staton and Maureen Martino, and posted on the *www.FiercePharma.com* website, CEO salaries for top pharmaceutical companies are listed. The CEO paychecks range from a low of $11.1 million for Bristol-Myers Squibb, to a high of $33.4 million per year salary for Abbott's CEO (Staton & Martino, 2008).

The Fact Sheet, 'Screening Mammograms,' from the National Cancer Institute, U.S. National Institutes of Health, concludes that the studies have not shown that having regular mammograms is of any benefit. Some studies show false negatives to occur – this is when mammograms appear normal when breast cancer is present, which often happens in younger women with dense breasts. They estimate up to twenty percent of all mammograms, miss breast cancers that are actually there (National Cancer Institute, 2010). Here: http://www.cancer.gov/cancertopics/factsheet/detection/mammograms

Other studies showed that false positives occur when women are diagnosed with cancer but none is actually present. Again, false positives occur more often in younger women with dense breasts. They also occur in women with family history or previous biopsies, or women on hormone replacement therapy (National Cancer Institute, 2010).

Just how many false positives are there? According to 'Predicting the Cumulative Risk of False-Positive Mammograms,' a study published in the *Journal of the National Cancer Institute*, "24% of the women had at least one false-positive mammogram. We estimated that the risk of a false-positive reading after ten mammograms was 49.1%" (Christiansen, Wang, Barton, Kreuter, Elmore, Gelfand et al., 2000).

What does that mean? It means that by the time a woman has had 10 mammograms, the chance of her being told her results are abnormal at some point, when they really aren't, are almost fifty percent.

In 'A Panel Discussion' (download), published online March 6, 2002, in Springer-Verlag, *Pediatric Radiology* (2002) 32: 242-244, Dr. Elaine Ron makes some interesting comments about the risk of cancers from radiation exposure. She explains, "in 50 years we have seen the lifetime effects of radiation, and we know what it can do to people. Radiation exposure from the atomic bomb at Hiroshima taught us that Leukemia is the first cancer to happen after radiation exposure, developing within 2 to 5 years after exposure, thyroid cancer develops next, about 5 years and solid cancers take longer, 10 or 20 years." Ron explains that it is concerning when children develop cancers from radiation exposure. When they have total body *irradiation* cancers can occur fairly soon (Springer-Verlag, 2002). Download here: http://www.springerlink.com/content/p1wwgcyddu2wqrjy/fulltext.pdf.

Surgery, radiation therapy, and chemotherapy are treatment options that may extend survival and/or relieve symptoms in many patients, but seldom produce a cure.

Cancer Facts & Figures, 2007.

HOW THE CANCER INDUSTRY CONTROLS WOMEN*

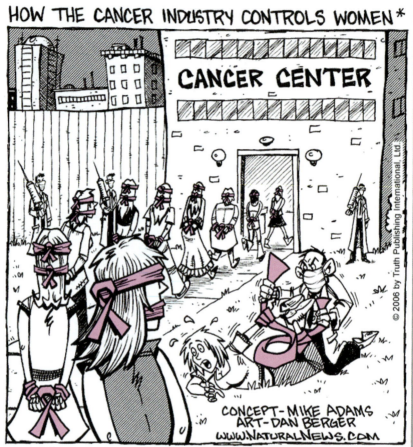

*FACT: Breast cancer screening harms ten times as many women as it helps.
See http://www.NaturalNews.com/020829.html

Mike Adams is the creator of the "Education, not Medication"
program that seeks to help women <u>prevent</u> breast cancer.

Reprint Courtesy: Cartoon created by Mike Adams of
www.NaturalNews.com.

18   Choosing Your Treatment

Cancer feeds on fear, and so does the industry that supports it. We are so afraid when faced with a diagnosis of cancer that we cannot see past fear to make rational decisions. Often, we are rushed through from diagnosis to mutilating treatments without enough time to pack an overnight bag.

If cancer took ten years to grow enough to be noticed, then surely we can take the time to discuss all of our options, with trusted practitioners, before we start removing body parts. It seems as though alternative options are something we consider only after we have let doctors take care of our illness. The problem is, it is not working. By the time many people decide to heal their body naturally, they have accumulated so much damage to their organs and systems it becomes very difficult to reverse the desecration.

Does this mean you should not have chemotherapy, radiation or surgery? In my opinion, this means you have to know that you *can* heal yourself without chemotherapy, radiation and surgery; without torturing yourself.

It is important to be aware of the benefits and drawbacks of any treatment you choose. One way to know if a therapy is beneficial is to ask some simple questions.

1.   What are the ingredients?
2.   Are they safe?
3.   Will it promote the health of my body or cause it to digress?
4.   What are the benefits?
5.   What are the side effects, adverse reactions and long term effects?
6.   Is there a natural solution that works just as well without temporary or permanent detrimental effects?

My personal experience has shown that some doctors tend to focus on adverse reactions, like nausea and hair loss, and leave out information about long term effects, such as liver, kidney or brain damage. Some pharmaceutical drugs can have far reaching and lifelong effects, causing permanent damage to vital organs, our immune system and the tissues of our bodies. Whether you are being subjected to radiation from a diagnostic tool such as a CT scan, bone scan, mammography or barium enema, or using a treatment tool such as surgery, chemotherapy or radiation, ask for the details of short and long term effects. Don't be shy. Be sure to take this list home with you so you can take your time thinking about and researching your options, without any pressure from outside forces.

If you cannot get answers to your questions from the person providing the treatment, then first of all, they should not be administering something they do not understand the consequences of, or provide full disclosure for, and second, searching the internet will provide ample knowledge about the drugs and treatments you are being offered.

Do not take anything, until you have become informed enough to make an educated decision, and be sure to look at *all* of the available evidence.

Do not rely solely on the opinion of the person administering the medication or treatment, even if you feel intimidated. Once you have collected and scrutinized all the information, then you can rely on your own decision to be the right one.

The same is true for natural therapies. Ask the same questions – they can also cause adverse reactions and side effects. In order to feel comfortable with any therapy or treatment, you must gather as much information as possible and make an informed decision and . . . that decision is ultimately yours.

Pay attention to your feelings and never make decisions about treatments when you are being pressured by someone else.

Are you with me?

Never make decisions about treatments when you are being pressured by someone else.

Thinking about the right path will make you feeeel better, while thinking about the wrong path will make you feeeel worse. Your body instinctively knows what it wants, and will tell you what to do, whether you are paying attention or not! Learn to recognize these feelings for the important messages they are relaying to you. You will recognize these feelings, if you stay aware.

It seems so simple, but when cancer patients are under pressure to agree to treatments, they are so stressed, they have no composure to ask even the simplest of questions. Becoming educated about the ingredients and effects of the treatments you are using is imperative to successful healing.

Choose therapies that are proven to work because people have used them and experienced their remarkable healing properties.

Be suspicious of treatments that are *proven* by a study which is funded by pharmaceutical or chemical companies.

Our most efficacious regimens are loaded with risks, side effects and practical problems; and after all the patients we have treated have paid the toll, only a minuscule percentage of them is paid off with an ephemeral period of tumoral regression and generally a partial one.

Edward G. Griffin, *World Without Cancer*, 2003.

19   Forcing Treatment

Whose choice is it?

It is your choice.

You have the right to choose which therapy you want, right?

Well, yes, and no! If you are a child, even your own parents cannot choose for you, even though, other than you, they are the people most likely to have your best interests in mind.

In May of 2008, an eleven year old Hamilton boy was taken from his family when he refused chemotherapy treatments, with his parents' support. Youth Protection Workers from the Canadian Children's Aid Society removed the child and placed him in foster care.

The boy was diagnosed with acute lymphoblastic leukemia when he was seven, at which time he underwent chemotherapy treatments. Too bad he did not have antifungal treatments like the nurse!

The cancer returned but neither the boy nor his family wanted to experience the grueling, dangerous treatments again.

Doctors said the boy would die in six months if he did not agree to chemotherapy. The courts ordered the boy to comply, and he was hospitalized and treated against his wishes (Brown, 2008).

Similarly, in the United States, in January of 2009, A thirteen year old boy, Daniel Hauser, was diagnosed with Hodgkins Lymphoma.

In February he underwent one chemotherapy treatment, but hated it so much he refused more. A Minnesota court ordered Daniel and his parents to seek the advice of an oncologist and have a chest x-ray taken (Adams, 2009).

The boy and his mother disappeared for a few days and authorities had a warrant for Daniel's mother's arrest. Out of fear, Daniel and his mother returned home (Adams, 2009).

We have learned that we are not alone in this quest to retain our parental rights and to insure that Danny has the opportunity to be cured from cancer and return to complete wellness and vitality.

Mrs. Colleen Hauser

Families are fighting to NOT receive medical treatment, because they know the treatment for cancer is worse than the disease itself!

Why are children being ripped away from their families and ordered to undergo dangerous chemotherapy treatments? These families know what they want and seem well informed about their situations.

Would you let a doctor take your child away and force poisonous treatments on them, against your own wishes and beliefs?

If Daniel Hauser was just three years older he would be able to refuse medical treatment. The age of medical consent in Canada is sixteen years of age and sixteen to eighteen years of age in most of the United States.

Clearly our laws need to be changed and medical doctors and child authorities need to stop forcing poisonous treatments on children, simply because they think they know better. No state ever has been, or ever will be, better at making decisions for our children than we are ourselves.

Mike Adams from Natural News updates us on Daniel's situation and the issues surrounding the horrendous forced poisoning of one of America's children.

Part One: 'Health Freedom and the forced chemotherapy of Daniel Hauser.' Here: http://www.youtube.com/watch?index=1&playnext=1&v=pFNMM1bDDK8&list=PL4AE732D1A4B2F9BA

Part Two: 'The forced chemotherapy of Daniel Hauser.' Here: http://www.youtube.com/watch?v=F84weZ6-Qu8&feature=related

What right do doctors and health authorities have to force toxic chemotherapy on Danny just because he is a child?

Don't they know he is sick?

No one should be able to take away the freedom to make our own health decisions. Maybe like Billy Best, Danny will really run away and cure himself.

Billy is now a thirty-one year old man, but at sixteen, he escaped from damaging chemotherapy treatments for Hodgkin's Lymphoma.

Doctors threatened that if Billy didn't have chemotherapy he would certainly die.

Well, Billy did not have chemotherapy and he did not die! Billy ran away, began eating roots, superfoods and medicinal herbs and drank Essiac tea, all of which cured his cancer. Now, fifteen years later Billy is alive and well, even though his doctors said he would be dead if he refused chemotherapy . . .

See Mike Adams's interview with Billy Best, 'Exclusive Interview with Billy Best, who Fled Chemotherapy at Age 16 and Beat Hodgkin's Lymphoma.' Here: http://www.naturalnews.com/026337_cancer_Billy_Best_chemotherapy.html

FORCING TREATMENT ON CHILDREN

CANADIAN BOY FORCED TO HAVE CANCER TREATMENTS

'Sick boy's family in court today' "They're fighting to get back 11-year-old taken by Children's Aid after refusing chemotherapy" (Brown, 2008, TheStar.com, http://www.thestar.com/article/424747)

DANIEL HAUSER – AMERICAN BOY FORCED TO HAVE CANCER TREATMENTS

'Daniel Hauser and the Side Effects of Cancer Treatments for Hodgkin's Disease'. 'Why did Daniel Hauser flee from Chemotherapy treatments?" (Adams, 2009, NaturalNews.com, http://www.naturalnews.com/026386_cancer_radiation_treatment.html)

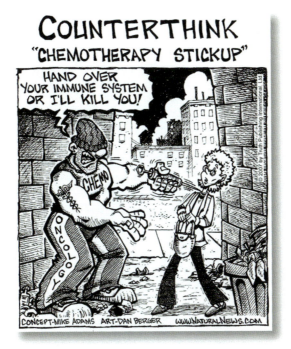

Reprint courtesy: Cartoon created by
Mike Adams of www.NaturalNews.com

Update on Daniel Hauser

In May of 2010, Daniel Hauser celebrated his fourteenth birthday *cancer free.*

Daniel's mother told Scott Wasserman, in a report by FoxTV, that Daniel is doing well on a strict sugar-free diet, with fruits and vegetables and very little meat. She reports that Daniel is doing whatever it takes to make sure his cancer does not reoccur. Here: http://www.myfoxtwincities.com/dpp/news/Daniel-Hauser-Turns-14,-Is-Cnacer-Free-mar-28-2010

Colleen, Daniel's mother is now facing stress from the large financial bills for Daniel's forced chemotherapy treatments (Wasserman, 2010).

Reasonable people adapt to the world. Unreasonable people persist in trying to adapt the world to themselves. Therefore, all progress depends on unreasonable people.

George Bernard Shaw

20 The Real Cure For Cancer

What have others done to cure themselves?

There are two common threads that run through all successful healings.

First, people who heal themselves are proactive, educated and in control.

Second, the choose natural therapies which create an environment inside their body that is conducive to health and inhospitable to cancer.

You can tell if natural therapies are working because they make you feel better! Feeling is important. To heal, you must be in tune with your body. Listen to the messages it gives you, and trust your inner awareness and gut feelings.

Natural therapies are soothing and supportive to a sick body, kind of like chamomile tea is to an upset stomach. They provide a balance of bioavailable nutrients, cleanse your organs and bodily fluids, improve immunity, keep pathogens in check and rebalance the pH of your blood, tissues and cells. They cleanse, heal and rebuild.

Many people claim to have found the cure to cancer, and to be honest, I feel a bit like that myself, after using my herbal tea on all kinds of large cysts, tumors, even melanoma; watching them dry up and peel away quickly and easily.

Can it really be this easy?

The truth is yes! Not only is it possible to cure cancer, it is downright simple.

As I learn more, I realize that there is only one cure for cancer and that cure was invented by no one.

Effective healing requires improved functioning of your immune system, detoxification of your body's tissues and fluids, and an abundance of vitamins, minerals, phytochemicals and other nutrients needed for killing invaders and repairing, protecting and rebuilding your cells, tissues and organs.

Your immune system uses immune cells to stop the growth of cancer. They are on constant guard, always searching for and destroying cancer cells, viruses and other invaders. A natural killer cell is one of the largest cells in your fluids and is monstrous in comparison to a tiny cancer cell.

When nourished properly, your immune system produces millions of cancer gobbling natural killer cells.

I know you can cure cancer with a Macrobiotic diet and Essiac™ tea; or you can cure cancer with a Vegan diet and burdock tea; or you can cure cancer by eating healthy, exercising and focusing your immune system, or you can cure cancerous tumors with a caustic escharotic and diet and lifestyle changes . . .

Natural Practitioners have really been saying the same thing all along. There is only one cure for cancer, but there are many ways to get there!

Well, if there is only one cure what is it?

Are you ready?

Drumroll please . . .

To heal yourself from anything, including cancer, just believe in your body's ability to heal itself; then give it the peace, love, food, herbs, water, air, sunshine, rest and joy it needs to do so!

Lisa Robbins, 2007.

21 More Treatments

It is 2006 and doctors talk my mother into chemotherapy treatments again.

Have they forgotten so fast, it almost killed her the first time?

We drive to Toronto to have a stunt put into her arm so the chemotherapy drug can be administered automatically, over several months.

The next day a nurse comes to my mother's house to attach the bottle of chemotherapy. Within 24 hours my mother is violently vomiting. The next morning she insists someone come back and remove the drug and stunt. They grudgingly oblige and send a nurse.

Four weeks later, after having only one 24-hour dose of chemotherapy, half of her hair falls out in huge clumps, over a one week period.

IN THE NEWS

In 'Doctors Urged to Stop Chemo,' the BBC explains why doctors are being urged to stop giving chemotherapy to sick people, stating that it caused or quickened death in 27% of cases! (BBC News Online. 1, 2008)

This next article highlights the drug my mother was given by her physician, in a study she agreed to take part in..

In 'Brain Damage Link to Cancer Drug,' authors show that the drug, 5-fluorouracil, referred to as 5-FU, in the article and on my mother's documents, is believed to cause brain damage, the effects lasting for 'years'. 5-fluorouracil is used to treat breast, ovarian, colon, stomach, pancreas and bladder cancers. The study concludes fluorouracil destroys "vital' cells in the brain involved with nerve function (BBC News Online. 2, 2008).

The majority of the cancer patients in this country die because of chemotherapy, which does not cure breast, colon or lung cancer. This has been documented for over a decade and nevertheless doctors still utilize chemotherapy to fight these tumors.

Levin, 1990.

68

22 Bitter Tonic Tea & Giant Cyst

In the Spring of 2007, I am at a baseball game with friends. I turn to talk to my friend Pat and notice a huge brown cyst on the side of her neck. "What the heck is that?," I ask.

She puts her hand up to feel it and says, "I have no idea, but it won't go away."

It's about the size of a large pea, dark brown, and kind of gross. "What about the tea?," I ask. "Do you want to try it?"

"Sure," she says."

The cyst is easily and safely removed with the tea. It shrinks and disappears. Nothing is left but beautiful, healthy, pink skin.

Several years ago I had a large, angry-looking cyst on the right side of my neck. It was sore, sometimes oozy, but it wouldn't go away. It was the size of a large pea. One night after playing baseball, Lisa recommended her anti-cancer herbal tea. Each night I soaked a cotton ball in the tea and taped it to my neck with hospital tape (bandaids left red marks on my skin). Within six weeks the cyst had shrunk and almost disappeared, so I kept using the tea for another month until all signs of the cyst were gone. The cyst has never returned and there is no mark or scar on my neck to this day.

Pat Lawson, June 2009.

23 Radiology Does Not Help

It seems like a while has gone by without any troubles for my mom, then in the late spring of 2007, we suddenly find ourselves back at the radiologist's office in Toronto. My mother is now seventy-four years old. The growth has *come back* in her right bronchi. She is coughing non-stop and is weak and tired.

We travel for one and a half hours from my mother's home, to the hospital where my father died twenty years before.

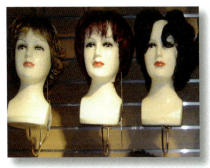

I feel the *cattle herding* aspect of the hospital immediately. Everywhere there are people with no hair, in wheelchairs, no colour in their faces, looking desperate and frightened. A huge shelf of sample wigs lays above the coat rack in the massive waiting room.

A nurse ushers my mother and I into a small clinic room. She asks my mother to take off her shirt and put on a hospital gown. I tie the back of the gown. We wait.

About forty-five minutes later a nurse comes in and tells us, the doctor will be with us shortly. A half hour goes by, then another half hour. I can only wonder, 'Why do we continue to sit here and wait? Are we that desperate for more bad news?'

Two hours and fifteen minutes after our appointment time the radiologist finally shows herself. She examines my mother. We are here to talk about the possibility of external radiation on the tumor in her bronchi. The doctor tells us that the growth is coming from her lung, growing through the outside wall into her bronchi tube.

This is news to us, after all this time. For years we believed the tumor started in her bronchi, not in her lung. I find a common thread of poor communication running throughout my mother's treatment.

At this point my mother is having considerable trouble breathing. The doctor tells her that if she doesn't have radiation, the tumor will continue to grow, blocking the bronchi. She will not be able to breathe, her lung will collapse and she will need oxygen. She is very sympathetic.

I look at the radiologist as she is sitting directly in front of both of us. We are both very upset about the whole situation. I say, "This is wrong. It is wrong that this is the only thing you can offer my mother. There are so many other things that we should be researching and trying. It is wrong that you can only offer her radiation or chemotherapy. You know there are other things."

She doesn't say anything. She continues trying to convince my mother that this is her only choice.

Later she looks at me and says, "You are right about what you are saying, but we don't have a choice."

My mother agrees to more radiation, even though I try to tell her it will make things worse, but . . . she is desperate.

The radiation does not help. It makes it extremely difficult for her to swallow. She grows progressively weaker and I begin to visit her daily. Gradually she becomes confined to her bed and only gets up to go to the bathroom.

I want to grow old.

Doris Elizabeth Dean, Spring 2007.

24 Another Friend Diagnosed with Breast Cancer

It is the summer of 2007. My friend Suzanne is diagnosed with breast cancer.

Suzanne took the contraceptive, Depo Provera for six months, two years before her diagnosis. One of it's serious adverse reactions is breast cancer. Is it possible she traded not getting her period for six months for breast cancer?

She was pre-menopausal and worried about heavy periods.

Unfortunately, no one took the time to discuss the many, many natural options for improving her hormone balance without taking dangerous synthetic hormones. And . . . no one ever thought to tell her that many women go through a period of heavy flow during menopause and that with most women, it will gradually wane and disappear, as she progresses through menopause.

A terrible lesson for us to learn at her expense: you are in charge of your own health and need to research everything.

She has two *massive* tumors buried deep inside her breast. She is not even fifty years old. Doctors completely remove her breast and all the lymph nodes in her armpit. They mention she may have some draining issues in her arm.

Fluid between cells is filtered and cleaned through her lymphatic system. The lymphatic vessels form a one-way flow of fluid through thousands of nodes. Proteins, cell debris, bacteria, viruses and cancer cells are normally prevented from entering her blood capillaries, but easily enter her permeable lymphatic capillaries, where they are pushed along through disease fighting nodes. Here lymphocytes examine, tag and destroy pathogens, cancer cells and debris (Marieb, 2003).

When women have all the lymph nodes cut out during breast removal, they most often have draining issues. Without lymph nodes, their hand and arm swells with fluid.

I have a friend who had the lymph nodes under her arm removed along with a melanoma that was situated on the top of her upper arm. She is forever holding her swollen arm and hand above her head, trying to drain the excess fluid.

The problem here is our misunderstanding of the function of a lymph node. This archaic thinking is based on the belief that lymph nodes should be removed so cancer cells cannot travel around the body through the lymphatic system.

Consider that the function of a lymph node is to house lymphocytes and cleanse the body of pathogens like bacteria, fungi, viruses and cancer cells. Lymphocytes are throughout your body, but you will find them concentrated inside lymph nodes. Here is where most of the immune work is done. Lymphocytes gobble up cancer cells.

If you remove your lymph nodes and their lymphocytes, how will they ever kill cancer cells for you?

I call Suzanne a couple of weeks after her surgery to see how she is doing. I warn her that doctors will want her to have bone scans, and try to tell her about the dangers. I am shocked when she tells me she already had one, and I am deeply saddened that doctors have already increased her risk for cancer occurring in her bones, before she has even recovered from having her breast removed.

25 Doctors Finally Manage to Kill My Mother

During the summer of 2007, my mother grows progressively weaker. By fall, she is admitted to palliative care for one week to "get her pain under control with proper meds," we are told.

For three days doctors tweak her medications until she is virtually pain free. I visit her regularly, and she seems to be doing very well. She is relieved that she is mostly pain free.

One afternoon, about one and a half weeks after she is admitted, I drop in to see her. No matter how hard I try, I cannot wake her up. She is unable to answer me or respond in any way.

I ask the nurse what is wrong with my mom, and wonder why she cannot talk to me. The nurse tells me in a comforting voice, "It is just the progression of her disease." She pats me comfortingly on the arm.

I respond, "I've been with my mother every day for this past year. This is not the normal progression of her disease."

My brother and I have to force nurses to give us a full list of my mother's medications, doses and frequency. Three times they give a list. The first list has medication names only. The second list includes doses. Finally, after asking a third time, we get the full list, including times the medications are given.

I immediately locate my friend who is a registered nurse. I am crying as I tell her, "My mom won't wake up, she can't answer me."

She looks at the list of medications. She is shocked at the strength of medications. "No wonder she can't wake up," she says.

She tells me what to delete and what to substitute. Medazolam is the drug that would not allow my mother to wake up. My brother and I have to force Power of Attorney before the doctor agrees to take my mother off Medazolam.

The next day my mom is fine again. For two months she lies in palliative care, waiting to die. Later she tells me, "They put me in a room by myself because they know I am dying. They are paying less and less attention to me."

I am silent. What can I say? I know it is true.

The food is repulsive, white pasta elbows with sticky, chemical-tasting, orange, cheese-like sauce, lifeless canned peaches, a slice of whole wheat bread, margarine and coffee. My mom hates coffee.

She is eating sugar like a maniac, a box of chocolates every three or four days. It seems very strange. It causes me to think back and remember my mother telling me about her Candida problems many years before and I realize that she has been fighting Candida her entire life. I remember her itchy ears and scalp, her bloated gut, her incessant craving for bread, and the chocolates . . .

I now realize, a simple fungus has killed my mother.

It's not *just* the fungus but more our lack of understanding. Our corrupt system treats sick people with poisons – massive overkill; while denying the primary problem of infection by a wee little fungus that is very simple to kill!

To think as a human race we value money over people. How pathetic.

The Candida has won. Now, I know the only thing I can do is help her to die.

After two months in palliative care, my mom *agrees* to go on Medazolam again. It knocks her out, and takes six days for her to die. It is sickening. On the fifth day I tell my brother, as I eye her pillow, "If she doesn't die soon, I'm going to kill her myself." I can't believe I am having such thoughts.

When she is clearly dying and there is no turning back, her doctor says to me, "Are you all right with what we are doing here?"

I just say, "Yes." I am beaten down, but I know in my heart of hearts what they are doing here; it is called euthanasia.

The nurses warn of imminent signs of death; they have seen it so many times before. Her knees will become blotchy and red. On day six of our vigil, I lift her sheet and jolt back when I realize their prediction.

They warn of a change in her breathing next. Several hours go by, then she takes a few short breaths and quietly slips away, leaving us behind in the dark, cold hospital room.

Before she died we often talked about the end. Not knowing what to expect, we were scared that cancer would consume

her body, choke off her airways, leaving her debilitated, gasping for breath, dying a terrible and painful death.

And yes, it was terrible and painful, but ironically cancer didn't kill her, her doctors did.

It's funny because for the last twenty years since my father died, I found it somewhat disturbing that he also didn't really die from cancer, even though that's what was supposed to have killed him.

Now I can honestly say, both of my parents were killed by cancer doctors and the conventional treatments used on them.

"

Lisa Robbins, 2008.

An Obsession

She was feisty and hard to put down . . . when I think of all she had been through I realize just how strong she had to be.

I hope my mother's death will be the end of my obsession with cancer but I begin to realize it has only started. I think about the secrets we learned together; which treatments can kill a person, and which therapies can heal a person.

I feel like her life was an experiment, not only for medical doctors, but for she and me as well. The more she did for herself, the better she became. The more conventional treatments she agreed to, the bigger toll they took on her poor worn out body and the worse she became.

Many people have wiped cancer from their lives without conventional treatments using harmless, safe and noninvasive therapies. They do not hurt your body, they heal your body.

How ridiculous to believe that poisonous chemotherapy will cure us or that cancer causing radiation will save us.

It reminds me of the primitive and dangerous procedure of bloodletting, which was used to treat U.S. President George Washington of a throat infection in 1799, but which experts believe, most probably succeeded in killing him (Wallenborn, 1997).

How many more precious lives will be squandered before we all *realize* and come to *know* the truth?

I work nights so I don't have to hang chemotherapy bags.

I hate it. I hate giving that shit to people. It's red poison going right into their bloodstream, right up into their brains.

I'm so sick of the medical industry. It's all about money, all of it.

April 2010, Fran B., Registered Nurse, Oncology, Canada.
Her name has been changed to protect her identity.

Alix my daughter introduced me to Fran in a grocery store, in the early winter of 2010, just over a month after Fran's mother had passed away. Alix and Fran had met a few years before when Alix was working in a cafe and had come to know each other fairly well.

Fran was visibly upset, was crying and did not hold back when she told us the truth about her job as an oncology nurse, and her mother's recent 'death from cancer treatments.'

She is speaking about the chemotherapy drug Adriamycin or Doxorubicin, nicknamed 'Red Devil,' after its dark red colour and dangerous side effects.

26 Toxic Waste

It is February of 2008, and my girlfriend Suzanne is being treated for breast cancer. Not long after her surgery, she is blasted with chemotherapy and radiation. Her hair falls out. She is an emotional wreck. She is down for months.

After her ordeal, she claims she will never again take chemotherapy. She says, "I feel like a walking toxic waste dump."

My research shows that chemotherapy was invented by Paul Ehrlich, who later became known as the 'Father of Chemotherapy.'

It's first application against cancer was in the 1950s. Some chemotherapeutic drugs are descended from the dangerous nitrogen mustards, used in World War II.

Six months after finishing chemotherapy for breast cancer, Suzanne's fingernails and toenails are falling off.

It is disgusting.

She says, "They told me to keep my toes and fingers in ice water during the chemotherapy treatments. I tried my best, but they fell out anyway."

She seems very sad and depressed.

27 Bag of Drugs

I fill a large bag with prescriptions from my mother's bedroom and handbag, everything from sleeping pills to laxatives, Tylenol 3's, antacids, Morphine and Prochlorazine for psychotic disorders, Celebrex, steroid inhalers, Paxil . . . wait a second, back up . . . psychotic disorder? I can't help but think, 'No wonder she's dead.'

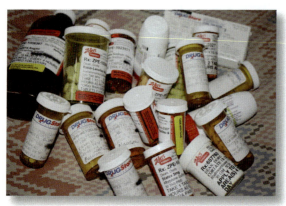

I am curious if the physicians who *cared* for my mother ever thought their mounds of drugs, radioactive scans and cancer causing chemotherapy and radiation treatments might have contributed to the spread of her cancer?

I sure do. My mom's father had bowel cancer too. Luckily for him though, he wasn't offered chemotherapy or radiation because it was only 1970. Doctors had not begun prescribing copious amounts of drugs yet. He had surgery only. Doctors removed the tumor and re-sectioned his bowel just like they did with my mother.

Interestingly, he did not die of cancer. When he was diagnosed with cancer he was seventy-three years old. Fifteen years later at the age of eighty-eight, he stood up from his couch, suffered a massive heart attack, and was dead before he hit the floor.

Do you think he did not die from *cancer* because he was not treated with cancer causing, toxic drugs and radiation?

28 Bitter Tonic Tea and Melanoma

This story is the raison d'etre of why I finally sat down and pieced this journal together. It was so visual and so confirming for me, that I knew I could not hold back this information any longer.

Roger, a kind and friendly man I know, has a nasty black melanoma growing down the back of his ear. His ear is literally being eaten away by the cancer.

Melanoma is the most dangerous skin cancer we are told. He tells me the cancer has been growing for about ten years. Ten years, I think? Seems like a long time for such a deadly cancer. Roger tells me doctors have scheduled surgery on his ear and radiation on his head to follow. He is not happy about the prospect of radiation treatments on his head. I ask Roger if he would join me in an experiment and he obliges willingly.

I mix up a fresh batch of tea and drop off a small dropper bottle. I am busy with other things and I forget about Roger for the next couple of weeks.

Two weeks later I am hosting a booth at our local home show and Roger and his wife come to see me there. He points to his ear saying, "That stuff you gave me is working."

"Pardon?" I say, not realizing what he is talking about right away.

"The tea you gave me is working, see?" he says again, pointing to his ear.

I can't believe my eyes. Over half that nasty black melanoma is gone. The ear is pink and healing beautifully underneath. Did you get that? In only two weeks, the deadly melanoma is over half gone.

It is hard to believe that something so simple can cure cancer, but that's only because the truth has been hidden from us for so long. Roger had a diagnosed melanoma, and the tea was causing it to disappear in days. The tea was applied by Q-tip for only two weeks before Roger's surgery so our experiment was cut short, but still, the results were amazing!

Roger sends me an email.

I just finished the tea. It seems to have worked best on the cancer on my ear. The cancer has not spread, nor has it reopened. The scab has become hard but it has not fallen off as yet. I go in to the cancer clinic on Thursday April 15th. We could not get a cotton soaked in the solution to adhere in a satisfactory manner, however. Donna coated the ear-infected area with a saturated Q-tip. She repeated this procedure 2-3 times a day. Many thanks for letting us try the tea. With a little more time, I think the cancer would have disappeared.

Roger Morningstar, April 2008.

29   A *Devine* Healing

Here is where things start to get really interesting . . .

It is June of 2008, and Linda Devine, a holistic coach and mentor, is diagnosed with breast cancer. At first, Linda is deeply disturbed and frightened, but with immeasurable courage she steps away from conventional treatments and chooses instead to heal her body naturally, using only simple diet and lifestyle changes.

What follows is an excerpt from the transcript of a personal interview with Linda in February of 2009.

Linda: *I went to a doctor and she found a tiny lump. They decided to do a mammogram which I wasn't really thrilled about but I thought, well, okay I'm going to do it. In the mammogram they did see something, so they did an ultrasound and then the doctor confirmed that it was definitely cancer and I should have surgery and then radiation. I asked him then about natural therapies and he just kind of laughed at me.*

Lisa: *You must have been scared.*

Linda: *I was very scared. I was so scared that I honestly didn't know what to do. I think it was worse because of their attitude, you know it was like, oh well, this is just routine, it's no big deal. You are just a number, not really a person, you know? The bedside manner was absolutely horrendous.*

Lisa: *Were you seeing an oncologist, or someone else?*

Linda: *Well, he made an appointment for me to see an oncologist and scheduled the surgery and the radiation, and when I left that office, I was in such a stupor, that I was just . . . just beside myself.*

Because, the very first thing you think is, Oh my God, I'm going to die, I'm going to die. Then when I really started to think about it, Okay wait a minute, it's only a little lump, they caught it really early, so maybe they can just remove the whole thing and it will be gone.

Then I started thinking, the cut and burn thing, that's just not me, that's not what I believe, and here, I've been advocating natural health and yet I'm considering to have this done? Then, I kind of got my head back and I decided, no, I'm not doing it.

Lisa: *Did you talk to them about that choice, or did you just not go back?*

Linda: *Oh, no, I talked to them, they tried to talk me out of it and basically my doctor fired me.*

Lisa: *So, let me just back up a minute. When you were diagnosed in that very first appointment, they were already booking surgery and radiation, right there?*

Linda: *Oh yeah.*

Lisa: *So, you were in shock.*

Linda: *I was in shock, I didn't have time to even think about it. He actually said to me that if he hadn't been so busy that day, they would have done it that day. They don't even want to give you a chance to think, and thank goodness, thank goodness, I had that time, because my appointment wasn't scheduled for another week.*

Lisa: *So what happened after the appointment?*

Linda: *I knew I couldn't drive, because I was just too shaken up. I walked home, and in that walk, that's when I decided. I'm not doing surgery, I'm not doing radiation.*

My body just told me, "No, it's the wrong thing to do."

Lisa: *But you already know a lot about natural healing.*

Linda: *Well, I would say enough, you know. Not as much as a lot of other people. I haven't taken any formal education or training, but I've done lots of research.*

It's a horrible situation to find yourself in, but once you get past that initial shock, and realize that you are the only person that can take responsibility for your own body, and it's not up to them, you know, YOU have to find out about what happens to your body.

If you really listen to your body, you know the right thing to do.

All the research I did guided me to exactly what I needed to see, what I needed to read, where I needed to go, everything.

Lisa: *Okay, now we are going to get to the big question. What changes, what supplements, diet changes, stress reduction, what things did you do?*

Linda: *I did some research around various diets and foods and what would be the best thing for me, again listening to my body. Probably about six or eight months previous, I'd started doing some research on Macrobiotic eating, and it's funny how your body leads you to things like that. I thought there was obviously a reason why I was already led to that, so I did more research on Macrobiotics and it just felt like the right thing, so that's what I did. I was really, really strict on myself, which is difficult for me because I absolutely love bread. So, no wheat, no gluten, no yeast, nothing like that. That was tough, but I did it.*

As far as supplements, I got hold of B17, which is Laetrile, and took that for about six months, and every once in a while I think, am I okay without it, and I'm just guided, and just listen, you know?

I also took Maitake.

Lisa: *Maitake mushrooms? What form did you take those in?*

Linda: *Well, a capsule, I actually took the Host Defense by New Chapters. That's a really good one. It's really difficult to get pure Maitake, without anything else in it, so there's various other mushrooms in it as well.*

I also took Zinactive, that's a prolithic enzyme. That was from the Naturopath who recommended I read the book, How to Prevent and Treat Cancer with

84

Natural Medicine by Dr. Michael Murray, and it's a really good book, so I would recommend that too.

There were so many things I was taking. Extra Vitamin C to bowel tolerance.

Vitamin D, I was walking outside quite a bit, so wasn't taking supplements when I was outside, but now that I can't get outside as much because of the winter weather, I'm taking a Vitamin D oil supplement. Omega 3, a really good multivitamin, Vitamin A, turmeric.

Some of the things I did were meditation and visualization. In one meditation I actually saw the cells being removed and I just observed, I didn't control it in any way.

Lisa: *How long did you meditate for?*

Linda: *Probably about four years on and off now. I'm not a religious meditator day by day, I don't do it that way, but when I feel I need it, I do it. I do meditate every day, but I may do five minutes or ten minutes, but not for hours.*

Lisa: *It's probably easy for you to get into that mode of meditation if you've practiced for that long.*

Linda: *Yes it is, and even though there's angst and there's panic and there's fear, you know that once you get into that meditative state, that all goes, and then you can focus on what's in there and what you need to do. So you can visualize where the cancer cells are, where the illness is, and that's how I guide people to what to do. To really just sit with it and be there, be there with whatever it is and then you can guide it to do whatever you need it to do.*

No negative TV shows.

Lots of sea vegetables, mostly organic whenever I could get them and whey protein too to help with glutathione in the liver.

Lisa: *I want to back up just a little bit and talk in more detail about the macrobiotic diet, because a lot of people don't understand what that is.*

Linda: Okay, sure. Basically macrobiotic diet is grains, greens and beans, so as long as you have about 40 to 50% of grains, about 40 to 50% green vegetables, and then 10 to 20% of beans and other things you can put into soup.

Miso soup is a big one on the list so I have it pretty much every day. Leafy greens that grow towards the sun are better. They really base their diet on the climate you live in. So here being a North American climate, leafy greens that point towards the sun are really good for our bodies because we are pulling that energy from the sun.

The grains, it's better than eating things like potatoes, and ground vegetables, things like peppers, tomatoes, the nightshades.

So about half whole grains, and half vegetables and local fruit, apples, things that grow in this North American climate. I stopped eating bananas, even though they are so rich in potassium. To bring things in that are grown in a completely different climate it just doesn't gel with what our bodies' need.

So they are very much into things that are grown in the same type of climate as we are in. For us that means swiss chard, kale, spinach, cabbage, apples, carrots and so on.

And it's the way you cook too, a lot of chopping and cutting. It's your frame of mind when you are preparing the food. It's a lot of yin and yang energy, that depends on what type of food it is and what kind of energy you need to cure the illness you have.

Lisa: What changes in attitude did you have?

Linda: It's really, really important to stay as positive as you can and it's hard to do because you're scared and you hope you're doing the right thing, and you have doubts about what you are doing. The key is to really stay positive and surround yourself with positive people.

If you've got a friend that is rather negative, just remove yourself from that person for a while.

Just focus on yourself, you really need to do that. Stay positive.

Lisa: *How do you know that your cancer is gone?*

Linda: *I feel it, and I confirmed it with thermography.*

Lisa: *So, in only ten months you not only cured your own breast cancer, but you brought yourself back to an excellent state of health. You really look great.*

Linda: *Yes, I cured my own cancer and I feel great as well, thank you.*

Lisa: *So what do you feel is the difference between your approach to healing cancer and someone who chooses conventional treatments?*

Linda: *Well, I am confident that natural therapies work and I think a lot of people are not quite that confident yet. I know people who believe in natural therapies and they go along with it. Then they are diagnosed with a life threatening illness and they let their doctor talk them into conventional treatments. I've seen people die from it.*

I know a man who developed pancreatic cancer and went for surgery and it just spread through his whole body.

What doesn't make sense to me is, why would you expose someone to something that is detrimental to their health when they're already sick? Why would you do that? That doesn't make any sense. When I hear about these things happening to people it's just heart wrenching.

Lisa: *If someone was diagnosed with cancer what would you tell them?*

Linda: *Do research, for your own good, do research. Stay as positive as you possibly can, I know it's hard, but stay as positive as you possibly can. Once you pass the initial shock it gets a little easier and a little easier.*

Find a support system. I met some awesome friends who I could talk to, and cry on their shoulder and scream at.

Have faith. Whether you call it God or the Creator or whatever you want to call it, there is a higher power out there, so have faith.

It's not meant to be for you to be sick. Everyone is meant to be healthy, but we need to take responsibility for our health. If you just allow others to do it to you, and follow their advice, that's not necessarily the best thing for your body.

Lisa: *So you have a chance to control your health and your future.*

Linda: *You do. You do.*

Lisa: *What about people who have not been diagnosed, but oftentimes we feel something is wrong and we are scared. What would you tell someone like that?*

Linda: *If they are the type of person who are really in tune with themselves, I would say meditate and ask, really get into that space, and ask if there is anything you should be concerned about, that you need to take care of. You will be guided to the right trail. Some people believe that macrobiotic cooking is not the right way, because they believe in a raw food diet. That's okay, for some people that's the way to go. You know the macrobiotic diet is not the answer for everyone.*

Lisa: *But it's certainly healthier than the diet most people are eating.*

Linda: *Oh my goodness, yes. Oh, absolutely.*

Lisa: *So, it's providing their body with the nutrients they've been needing.*

Linda: *Well, exactly. It's taking away all of that junk food. That's the primary thing. That's what people need to get rid of. Stop going to fast food places. You know you're eating burgers with heaven only knows what's in them, and french fries, and bags of potato chips. That's garbage for your body. It's horrible stuff.*

Lisa: So not only are you filling your body with chemicals and trans fats, but you're depriving your body of the nutrients it needs to protect itself. That's the main problem. When you say you added sea vegetables, that's probably the best thing you could have done for yourself, is to add those rich nutrients back into your diet from sea vegetables.

Linda: There's one dish that I make with Daikon radish that is a little bit strange. I grate Daikon and grate a whole carrot and boil that and one umeboshi plum chopped in little pieces, and I take a piece of Nori, the seaweed they use to wrap around sushi. I take that and its like a soup and its really good for reducing tumor growth and so many other things.

That's the thing when you start eating healthy, healthy foods do so many good things for your body, not just one thing.

You have so much more energy, and it's the clarity too. There are many other things out there that are equally as good but this is what suited me.

There's a really good recipe with Daikon, and Lotus Root and Cucumber. That's really good too, in the summer.

Lisa: What kinds of cleanses did you do?

Linda: The macrobiotic diet is kind of a cleanse in itself, but I started on an Isagenix program which is shakes with whey protein. The whey protein that is in their product, is not denatured and it hasn't been exposed to any pesticides or any kind of pharmaceuticals. They get it from cows in New Zealand, and they aren't exposed to pesticides, they aren't injected with hormones or anything like that. It's the purest form of whey protein that you can possibly get, and that's what I'm looking for.

They also have a product that's called Ionic Supreme that has about 200 nutrients in it, so a shot of that a day. I started in October, so a couple of months.

89

It's expensive, but you know what, it's your health, and when you are dealing with your health, it's worth it.

Lisa: I feel that the gist of what you are saying, is that regardless of what way you choose, whether you choose a raw diet, whether you choose an herbal tea that cures cancer, or you choose a macrobiotic diet, which many others have used to cure cancer, or whether you choose to take garlic therapeutically, if it's something that will help your body, as opposed to something that will hinder your body's ability to heal, that's the better choice.

Even mammograms . . .

Linda: Yes, it's radiation going into your body.

Lisa: It definitely causes breast cancer. There's no doubt about it. So, not just the treatments, but even the tools used to diagnose breast cancer, cause it themselves.

Linda: Thermography doesn't harm in any way. The more we make people realize what the options are, what is available, that you don't have to do the cut and burn, you don't have to, its just not necessary, then we can make intelligent decisions, based on what we know.

Lisa: Are there any resources that you would suggest that people refer to if they are dealing with cancer?

Linda: There's a lot of information on the internet, but I would caution people to not take everything seriously that you read on the internet. Make sure you know what the source is, where it's coming from, because anybody can write anything on the internet, so just be careful where its coming from. One book that is very, very good is How to Prevent and Treat Cancer with Natural Medicine by Michael Murray. He is a doctor and a naturopath.

There are numerous other ones. I've probably read most of Michio Kushi's books, all on macrobiotics and healing. There are lots of case studies in his books, that outline the treatment that was given to people with lung cancer, cured; people with liver *cancer, cured; all kinds, skin cancer, and worse, much worse cases than what I've had.*

So, you know, it can be done. Absolutely, with no question.

Lisa: *What is most important for people to know?*

Linda: *I think the most important thing is to listen to your body and take responsibility for it. That's the biggest thing. It's huge, because there are just too many people that go to their doctor and say I'm sick, fix me. Well, they're not gods, they're not gods. They are normal people just like we are and they don't know. They don't know what the cure for cancer is.*

In April, two months after our interview, another thermographic exam of Linda's breast shows no sign of cancer present. After only ten months, Linda has cured her own breast cancer with diet and lifestyle changes!

Like others before her who have cured themselves, Linda applied the 10 Key Principles of Healing. Later I'll outline just what those ten key principles are.

Now Linda uses the experience of curing herself to help others through seminars and presentations such as *Healing From Cancer Naturally*. Her presentation summarizes her experiences with breast cancer and discloses, in detail, what steps she took to cure herself.

Linda is a dedicated healer who works endlessly to bring hope to others with joy, intelligence and enthusiasm. Through her own website at LindaDevine.com.

Linda was a speaker at *SpeakersFromTheHeart.com* where she spoke of her experiences healing breast cancer in her presentation *Healing From Cancer Naturally*.

30 Magnesium Deficiency

Inadequate levels of magnesium are known to increase the risk of cancer in your body.

You can safely assume that adequate levels of magnesium will protect you from cancerous growths, because this is exactly the case.

On the *Magnesium For Life* website, author of 'Transdermal Magnesium Therapy,' Mark Sircus, Ac., O.M.D. writes in *Magnesium And Cancer Research,* "Magnesium deficiency can lead directly to cancer . . . It is involved as a catalyst in over 300 enzyme systems; protects our cells from aluminum, mercury, lead, cadmium, beryllium and nickel; is essential for the synthesis of the most important antioxidant in the human body, glutathione," (we will learn more about this important compound soon); "is involved in cell membrane integrity; maintains the gradient of sodium and potassium inside and outside every cell in our body; and stabilizes ATP, allowing DNA and RNA transcriptions and repairs" (Sircus, 2010).

Magnesium is deeply connected to calcium in our bodies. Sircus states, "Magnesium deficiency poses a direct threat to the health of our cells. Without sufficient amounts, our cells calcify and rot. Breeding grounds for yeast and fungi colonies they become, invaders all too ready to strangle our life force and kill us" (Sircus, 2010).

MAGNESIUM – ARE YOU GETTING ENOUGH?

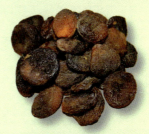

Magnesium is one of the most important nutrients cancer patients are missing and one of the easiest to get back into your body.

Symptoms of magnesium deficiency include insomnia, irritability, muscle cramps, twitches, spasms or tremors, gall stones, chocolate cravings, irregular heartbeat, excess body odor and cancer.

Eat magnesium rich foods everyday, such as almonds, and naturally dried apricots. Also rich in magnesium: raw fruits, vegetables, sea vegetables, dark chocolate, raw nuts and seeds.

Epsom salts (pure magnesium sulphate) are also a great source of magnesium. Most health foods stores or drug stores sell bags of salts to scoop into your bath.

Use half to one cup Epsom salts in a bath, to replenish magnesium levels in your body, and to feel calm and relaxed.

High calcium levels, on the other hand, have been shown to **increase** the risk of cancers, particularly prostate cancer. Several Harvard School of Public Health studies have shown high dairy intake was responsible for large increases in prostate cancer risk, and in some cases doubled or quadrupled the risk of metastasized prostate cancer (Sircus, 2010).

Animal studies show that magnesium deficiency caused convulsions and death in some infant rats, cardiorenal lesions in surviving rats and nodules on the thymus gland or lymphosarcoma on others (Bois, 1964).

Magnesium is so important that when magnesium-deficient rats had their levels replenished, it produced rapid disappearance of their periosteal tumors.

Hunt & Belanger, 1972.
Periosteal means in cartilage, attached to bone.

31 Bitter Tonic Tea™

It is June of 2009. We have tried the tea on everything, and there is nothing it does not get rid of. We have tried it on moles, boils, cysts, a diagnosed melanoma, basal cell carcinomas, even metastasized lung tumors.

The tea has proven to be an extremely strong ally in the fight against cancer, both externally and internally. We have seen it kill cancer cells quickly, while tissue repair takes place simultaneously, on external cancers and growths.

The combination of herbs in this blend provides an abundance of minerals, vitamins, phytochemicals, and anti-cancer properties, capable of changing the metabolic state of your body when taken internally. Our bodies need a rich pool of nutrients to pull from, to cleanse and to rebuild with healthy cells and tissues. These revitalized, healthy cells will be strong and more able to defend themselves.

In Dr. Duke's *Phytochemical and Ethnobotanical Database*, you can search any of the herbs in Bitter Tonic Tea™, and see the long lists of natural cancer fighting compounds, including alkalizing minerals, and lots of magnesium!

The chemicals are anything from Vitamin C to Arctigenin, a chemical found in the herb burdock, which, among other things, exhibits antileukemic, antilymphomic, anti-tumor, anti-tumor (liver), immunomodulator and immunostimulant properties.

If this database, created by the famous Dr. James Duke, lists thousands of anti-cancer properties in our herbs and plants, why are they not being used everywhere to fight cancer?

How is it possible that cancer patients are allowed to be treated with isolated extracts of plants, but are not allowed to be treated with the plants themselves, using traditional methods?

It seems ludicrous!

Native Americans learned the anti-cancer properties of herbs early on. Poultices and other preparations of effective herbs were applied externally and tea was taken internally to rid the body of cancers.

The most amazing thing of all is that herbal teas are healing medicines . . . not cancer causing poisons. An easily accessible, economically feasible, cancer killing, healing, herbal tea. It is so incredible, I have a hard time believing it myself sometimes . . . until I see it heal another growth . . .

Each of the herbs in the tea have strong healing properties. Knowing these properties can help you tweak the formula for yourself. For instance, if the tea acts too powerfully on your bowels, you can reduce the amount of Cascara Sagrada.

You can add other herbs like Chamomile, Rosemary or Lemon Balm for their comforting and calming properties.

If there are other herbs with specific properties you would like to add to your mixture, consult a master herbalist first to be sure there are no contraindications with the other herbs, with any medications you may be taking, or with your present condition, such as pregnancy or high blood pressure. A good herbal book can give you information about your herb, its characteristics, and applications.

When you are sure the herb is safe to add to the formula, go ahead and mix it in your blend. Now . . . it is *your* anti-cancer tea!

Other Names: Berberis vulgaris, Jaundice Berry, Barberry Root, Pepperidge Bush.

Parts Used: Bark of stem, leaves, roots and berries in fall.

Substitutions: Oregon Grape Root.

Properties: Antibacterial, antiviral, astringent, hypoglycemic, cholagogue (increases flow of bile), choleretic (stimulates excretion of bile by liver), depurative (purifies blood and lymph fluids), immunostimulant, prophylactic (contributes to the prevention of infection and disease), laxative, nutritive, remineralizing.

Indications: Liver and gallbladder disorders, painful periods and labour pains, jaundice, weakened or debilitated conditions, eye infections.

Considered invasive, Common Barberry is on U.S. and Canadian noxious weed lists. It is controlled near grain crops like oats, wheat, rye and barley, to protect them from Stem Rust Fungus, which overwinters on infested barberry leaves and causes infestations in spring grain crops (Ontario Ministry of Agriculture, 2003).

You will find Berberis vulgaris growing in the natural gardens at the Royal Botanical Gardens on the West shore of Lake Ontario. It is not native to North America, but did naturalize here, and can be found growing wild along road sides, riverbanks and the edge of forests throughout Southern Ontario (Ontario Ministry of Agriculture, 2003).

COMMON BARBERRY

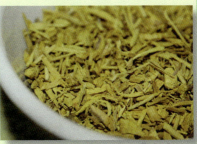

Dried root
Note characteristic yellow color

Like all the other Bitter Tonic Tea herbs, Berberis vulgaris, can be used on its own, as a *Simple* for specific effects, or can be mixed with other herbs for compound effects.

To make barberry tea, put one teaspoon of dried bark in a cup of cold water, bring to the boil, remove from heat and let steep at least 20 minutes.

For liver or gallbladder congestion, take 3 cups of tea daily, until symptoms are reduced and relief is achieved.

Use as mouthwash for mouth ulcers.

Drink 1 cup before meals for stomach ulcers.

I cannot ever remember seeing one growing in the wild in southern Ontario, but I do remember my grandmother's thorny barberry bush in northwest Toronto, when I was growing up.

It grows commonly in North American, European and Asian countries, and the bark and leaves are easy to buy in dried form, from herbalists and health food stores.

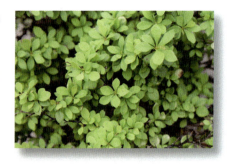

Common Berberis Bush, a smaller species, with tiny leaves and small red berries.

It has an upright growing habit and reaches up to ten feet, more like a tree than a shrub. It produces clusters of hanging pale-yellow flowers, and oblong red berries, which native bird species are very fond of. It has sparse, sharp thorns and characteristic yellow wood (Ontario Ministry of Agriculture, 2003).

Like many medicinal herbs, Common Barberry is poisonous in large quantities and medicinal in small amounts. It's active components are berberine, oxyacanthine and columbamine, all strongly antibacterial (Mabey, 1988).

The plant is a rich source of minerals, including calcium, phosphorous, magnesium, manganese and potassium, and tea made from the roots helps to remineralize your tissues and bones.

If you are lucky enough to own a common barberry, or know someone who does, pare the bark off the stems and unearthed roots in the early spring or late fall, and dry the roots and barks in the shade.

Like all the other Bitter Tonic Tea herbs, Berberis vulgaris, can be used on its own for specific effects. It's actions are laxative, bitter-tonic, anti-bilious, hepatic and anti-emetic (Hoffman, 1996).

The ground yellow rhizome stimulates bile flow, expelling gallstones, easing inflammation and congestion of your liver, improving digestion, detoxifying and purifying your blood and lymphatic systems. This makes it useful in acute hepatitis and jaundiced conditions.

It is also used to strengthen the system of weak, debilitated patients, and has been used to treat malaria, cholera and protozoal infections.

The rhizomes or roots of the Oregon Grape Root can be substituted for Common Barberry. This is because it contains the same alkaloid, berberine, so is useful in conditions where liver and gall bladder function need improvement and in arthritis and cancer (Hoffman, 1996).

The name Jaundice berry and the yellow color of its bark, another one of nature's messages, indicate its use in liver and gall bladder conditions . . .

Warnings:
Barberry is poisonous in large quantities, pay attention to dose.

Pregnant women should not use Barberry because of its stimulating action on uterine muscles.

Should not be taken for prolonged periods in preexisting conditions of anemia and hypothyroid (Tierra, 1998).

Burdock

Other Names: Arctium lappa, Common Burdock, Great Burdock, Greater Burdock, Burr, Gobo, Beggar's Buttons, Stick Button, Turkey Burrseed, Hareburr, Bardane, Cocklebur, Clotbur, Batweed, Love Leaves, Philanthropos (friend of man), The Herb of Ringworm Sufferer's.

Parts Used: All parts, root, leaves, flowers, seeds.

Properties: Depurative (purifies blood and lymph fluids), antibacterial, antiviral, astringent, hemostatic (stops bleeding), cholagogue (increases flow of bile), choleretic (stimulates excretion of bile by liver), hypoglycemic, immunostimulant, prophylactic (contributes to the prevention of infection and disease), nutritive, remineralizing.

Indications: Acne, arthritis, burns, constipation, eczema, gastrointestinal disorders, psoriasis, rheumatism, skin disorders.

Of all the names for Burdock, Beggar's Buttons is my favorite. It's flowers mature to burrs, the spiky seed heads well known for sticking to fur and clothing and whose structure was the inspiration for Velcro™.

Burdock is a large plant, reaching up to six feet. It grows prolifically in farm fields and in poor or sandy soil. The large tap

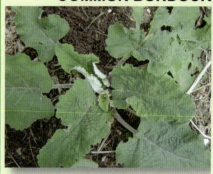

COMMON BURDOCK

Early growth, no flowers yet Spring, Southern Ontario, Canada

Leaves are perfect for picking and drying in this photo. In the fall dig up the root, wash, chop and dry. Leave some plants for next year to harvest flowers and seeds.

Make an infusion of Burdock root to assist in cleansing the body, by mashing 2 teaspoons of dried burdock root in a mortar and pestle. Place in a self-straining teapot, pour boiling water over and let the tea steep for 10 to 20 minutes. Drink one to two cups per day.

Make a more gentle form of tea by steeping one or two fresh leaves in boiling water and drinking. To ease skin eruptions of any kind, including acne, boils, psoriasis or eczema, soak a folded piece of cotton flannel in warm tea (made from leaves or roots), gently press to affected area, and leave for a while; or, mash the leaves and apply directly to the affected area.

root grows down almost as tall as the plant grows high, and is a staple root vegetable in Japanese cuisine, called *Gobo*.

Burdock grows wild in the fields surrounding my home in Southern Ontario. A few years ago it made its way into my garden. My girlfriend, a native of Canada, told me when a wild plant grows near you, it is because you need its medicine. I wonder if the burdock is trying to tell me something!

Burdock is the principle ingredient in my formula, as well as in both Rene Caisse's and Harry Hoxsey's original formulas.

All parts of the Burdock plant, including the leaves, roots, flower heads and seeds, have blood cleansing effects, which is why it is used against cancer, in herbal salves and teas. All parts have laxative, mild diuretic and sweat-inducing properties (Mabey, 1988).

> **CHAI BURDOCK TEA**
>
> Add a *masala* (spice mixture) to 2 or 3 teaspoons of burdock root in the teapot: 1 teaspoon cinnamon, 1 teaspoon ginger and half a teaspoon nutmeg.
>
> Add fresh creamy, nut milk – *Hemp Milk and other easy Seed and Nut Milks*. Here: http://thegoodwitch.ca/hemp-milk/
>
> Drink regularly for blood cleansing, supportive nutrition and anti-cancer benefits.

Burdock is one of the best known and longest used of the blood-cleansing herbs. It gently urges the body toward alkalinity by assisting the kidneys in removing uric acid, and is recommended for gout, arthritis, kidney and bladder infections. Burdock is helpful against chronic blood and skin diseases. It's bitter components stimulate your liver and gallbladder to secrete bile, greatly enhancing digestion and nutrient absorption. It possesses polyacetylenes which give the plant it's strong anti-microbial properties (Mabey, 1988).

Burdock provides an excellent cleansing remedy with depurative qualities. It removes the buildup of toxins and heavy metals, responsible for causing skin problems, arthritic and joint pain and digestive sluggishness. The leaves make a useful poultice for eczema, psoriasis, acne and skin disorders of any kind. Burdock is not only an excellent cleansing plant, it is also a rich source of valuable vitamins, minerals, carbohydrates, protein and fiber.

Burdock should be used gently, over several weeks or months, to assist your body to return to a state of balance.

In the summer of 2009, Shadow cured himself by eating burdock leaves.

He had an infection in his frog from stepping on a nail. That's the soft, fleshy part underneath his hoof.

The infection was quickly moving up his leg, and Shadow was not feeling well, so David let Shadow out to pasture.

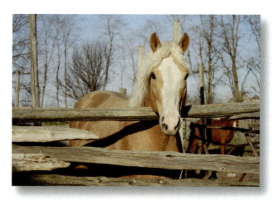

This is Shadow, isn't he beautiful?
That's his baby, Star, in the background.

Horses are very smart about what cures them, and he instinctively knew what to eat. He systematically stripped the leaves from every burdock plant in the pasture.

I asked David what he was doing because horses don't normally eat Burdock, even when they are hungry. He let out a big laugh and said, 'He's healing himself!' Sure enough, within days the swelling in his lower leg subsided and his frog was healing nicely.

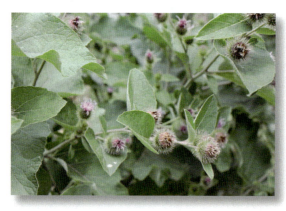

Burdock late summer, burrs forming
out of flowers

Another Burdock story . . . My friend, Mattie, told me about using burdock as a teenager, over 35 years ago. She had bad acne so her grandmother gave her a bottle of *Burdock Bitters*.

She drank the bottle as prescribed over a short period and has never had acne since.

Cascara Sagrada

Other Names: Rhamnus Purshiana, Cascara Sagrada, Chittem Bark, Sacred Bark, California Buckthorn, Purging Buckthorn, Bearberry, Holy Bark, Wahoo

Parts Used: Dried, aged bark

Substitutions: Buckthorn Bark, *Rhamnus Catharticus,* other species of buckthorn

Properties: Cathartic (produces bowel movements), antibacterial, antiviral, astringent, hemostatic (stops bleeding), cholagogue (increases flow of bile), choleretic (stimulates excretion of bile by liver), hypoglycemic, depurative (purifies blood and lymph fluids), immunostimulant, stimulant laxative, lithotriptic (dissolves stones), nervine (calms the nervous system), nutritive, purgative (produces bowel movements), remineralizing.

Indications: Chronic constipation, hemorrhoids, kidney and bladder stones, liver and gallbladder stones, liver congestion.

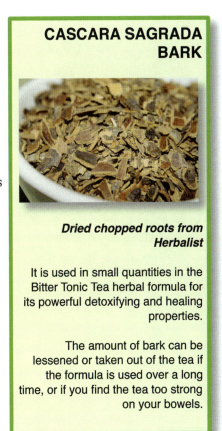

CASCARA SAGRADA BARK

Dried chopped roots from Herbalist

It is used in small quantities in the Bitter Tonic Tea herbal formula for its powerful detoxifying and healing properties.

The amount of bark can be lessened or taken out of the tea if the formula is used over a long time, or if you find the tea too strong on your bowels.

This tree is native to the northwest coast, growing from California to British Columbia. Cascara Sagrada, meaning Sacred Bark, was highly valued by the Algonquins, and other American natives, and was added to the *USP, United States Pharmacopeia* in 1890 (Vogel, 1970).

Cascara is known best for its laxative action, which increases bile flow and promotes intestinal peristalsis, the rhythmic contractions which move waste through your intestines. Though it has a fairly mild purging action, and rarely produces diarrhea, it should be used with caution (Tierra, 1998).

It was used traditionally by the Cherokee Indians of North America as a treatment for upset stomach and constipation, and as a remedy for itching and eye infections (Reader's Digest, 1998).

You will find Cascara Sagrada in laxative formulas in pill, liquid or powder form.

Warnings:
Cascara Sagrada should be avoided by pregnant and nursing women, small children, and people with stomach ulcers or irritable bowel syndrome.

Cascara is not normally used as a Simple, an herb used by itself, because it can cause cramping if taken alone or in excess.

Cascara should not be used for a lengthened period of time. Overuse of any purgative can cause longterm mineral loss, irritation to the mucous membranes of your intestines, and dependency on laxatives for elimination.

Cascara Sagrada or Buckthorn Bark can cause irritation to the lining of the intestines, and for this reason should not be used for more than three weeks without a doctor's supervision.

Irritation can be lessened by adding Slippery Elm, Chamomile or Fennel.

If your formula causes 'griping' pains, it may have too much Cascara Sagrada. Use less next time, or add ginger root to counteract this side effect.

Licorice Root

Other Names: Glycyrrhiza glabra, Glycyrrhiza Lepidote

Parts Used: Chopped or powdered, dried roots.

Properties: Adaptogen (adapts the body stress and reduces its effects), alterative (deep cleanser), antiallergic, anti-anemia, anti-arthritis, anti-estrogenic, anti-inflammatory, anti-microbial, anti-ulcer, anti-viral, demulcent (soothes and softens), expectorant (promotes clearance of mucous from respiratory tract), neutralizes toxins, fever reducing.

Indications: Adrenal gland problems, bronchitis, coughs, catarrh, respiratory tract conditions, stomach and duodenal ulcers, sore throat, sharp or intense pain.

The root of the Licorice plant is used as a natural sweetener. Chew on a piece of root, slowly at first, letting the enzymes in your saliva soften the root and release its sugars and medicinal properties.

Soothing and sweet, it is useful for gastric ulcers, sore throats and is helpful in reducing sharp or intense pain (Reader's Digest, 1998).

LICORICE ROOT TEA

Sliced, dried roots from herbalist

Licorice is one of my favorite herbs – it tastes delicious and is sweeter than sugar, up to fifty times sweeter!

You can make licorice tea on it's own. It is wonderfully soothing for strep or a sore throat of any kind, and it's adaptogenic properties make it an excellent stress fighter!

Add unpasteurized honey and fresh squeezed lemon juice to licorice tea for sore throats, colds and flus.

Licorice root tea:
1 teaspoon of dried, powdered root in 1 cup of boiling water. Steep 10 to 20 minutes. Drink 1 cup, 3 times per day.

See the Warning about overconsumption of Licorice and high blood pressure.

Licorice is one of the most widely used alterative herbs in the *Oriental Materia Medica*. Chinese use it to bring the body from a negative state to a healthy one (Buchman, 1996). Chinese call Licorice the 'great detoxifier', because it is known to drive poisons from the body (Ody, 1993).

104

Licorice has been used topically to treat skin conditions like psoriasis, eczema and allergic dermatitis and is considered equal to or superior to hydrocortisone cream (Duke, 1997).

To try this yourself, soak a folded cotton flannel or cloth in cooled licorice root tea and lay on the affected area. Leave for twenty minutes or more if possible. Repeat three or four times per day, until the condition is healed.

According to James Duke, Licorice contains "at least 25 fungicidal compounds, more than any other herb listed" (Dr. Duke's *Phytochemical and Ethnobotanical Database*, 1998).

Perhaps this is why it is so helpful in fighting cancer!

It is a balancing herb, used in herbal blends for its appealing flavor, reducing bitter flavors and enhancing the activities of herbs it is mixed with.

Licorice root is an adaptogen, a plant that increases the body's ability to handle stress. It works gently by assisting the immune system and the glandular system, in particular the stressed out adrenal glands, to relax the body and replenish it's vital energy.

It is recommended for infections in the lungs and respiratory passages, to loosen phlegm and make it easier to expectorate. Licorice root is used by itself in a *Simple* remedy or in herbal blends, for dry cough, bronchial congestion, hoarseness, wheezing and shortness of breath. *Simple* remedies use only one herb.

Licorice root is used in stomach ulcer therapy, for it's antimicrobial and soothing properties. In *The New Age Herbalist*, Richard Mabey states, "Licorice has a remarkable power to heal stomach ulcers because it spreads a protective gel over the stomach wall, and in addition, it eases spasms of the large intestine" (Mabey, 1988).

Wild licorice is a perennial plant, growing all over North America, from Mexico to Canada, and many other parts of the world. Native peoples chewed the fresh root to relieve toothaches and drank root tea to reduce fevers.

Licorice should never be eaten in large quantities, whether in it's natural, medicinal state, or made into tea or candy; see warnings.

Warnings:

In *large* amounts, licorice root can cause high blood pressure, salt and water retention and low potassium levels. Consult a physician if you take diuretics or water pills, or other medications that affect potassium levels, or if you have heart disease, high blood pressure, liver or kidney disease; before using licorice regularly.

Pregnant women should not consume large amounts of licorice in food or supplement form as it can increase the risk of preterm labor, due to it's hormonal activities (Reader's Digest, 1998).

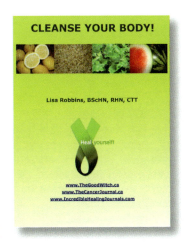

A note about skin conditions:

Skin conditions such as Psoriasis, Eczema and Allergic Dermatitis, can be addressed by liver and blood cleanses, and improvements in diet.

Download 'Cleanse Your Body' and start healing right now. Here: http://thegoodwitch.ca/start-with-cleanses-first/

Pau D'Arco

Other Names: Tabebuia Impetiginosa, Tabebuia Heptaphylla, Lapacho, Purple Lapacho, Tabebuia, Taheebo

Parts Used: Aged inner bark

Properties: Alterative (deep cleanser), anti-fungal, anti-cancer, hypotensive (lowers blood pressure), anti-diabetic, bitter tonic (bitter tasting medicine that increases strength and tone, stimulates appetite, improves digestion, and works to detoxify, cleanse and nourish tissues and fluids), digestive, antibacterial, anti-tumor.

Indications: Fungal infections, cancer, to slow and inhibit tumor growth, skin diseases.

Pau D'Arco is a tree, growing in the southern rain forests of Brazil and Argentina.

The quinone compounds of Pau D'Arco have been studied extensively for their potential use in pharmaceutical agents for cancer treatment. It has been used for thousands of years by natural healers and Native Indians in Latin America, to inhibit and slow the growth of cancers and tumors. Records of the Calaways, a tribe descended from the Incas, show they used Lapacho bark to treat cancer and many other diseases (Tierra, 1998).

PAU D'ARCO

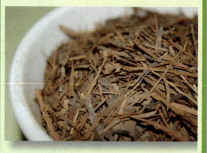

Dried inner bark

Buy quality Pau D'Arco. Some suppliers substitute outer for inner bark, or immature bark, which does not contain the same levels of cancer-fighting compounds.

Pau D'Arco makes a mild tasting, but potent healing tea. Use as a simple or blend with Red Clover and Burdock, for a blood cleansing, hormone balancing, cancer fighting powerhouse!

Simmer 3 tablespoons in a small saucepan of boiling water for 3 or 4 minutes. Remove from heat, cover and let steep for at least 20 minutes. Drink one cup of tea, 3 times per day.

Michael Tierra recommends a blend of Red Clover, Burdock, Chaparral, and Pau D'Arco tea for cancer. He suggests using equal parts of each herb, in water, three times per day. He reports in 1960, doctors at the Municipal Hospital of Santo Andre used an herbal preparation made from the bark of Pau D'Arco. The doctors reported, within thirty days, most patients no longer experienced pain, and many tumors were completely gone, or largely diminished. Tierra states, "Dr. Theodore Meyer of Argentina reported five leukemia victims, completely cured by Pau D'Arco. The herb is reportedly used in hospitals and clinics in South America to treat leukemia and other pathogenic diseases" (Tierra, 1998).

Listed below are the activities of Lapachol, the active quinone in Pau D'Arco, from Dr. Duke's *Ethnobotanical and Phytochemical Database*.
LAPACHOL *Bark*:
Antiabscess; Antibacterial; Anticarcinomic 100-400 ppm; Antiedemic; Antiinflammatory; Antimalarial; Antiseptic; Anti-Tumor; Antiviral; Fungicide; Immunostimulant 0.01 mg/ml; Insectifuge; Pesticide; Protisticide; Respiradepressant; Schistosomicide; Termiticide (Dr. Duke's *Phytochemical and Ethnobotanical Database*, 1998).

In *The Green Pharmacy*, Dr. Duke reports Lapachol bark contains lapachol, beta-lapachone and xyloidine, three compounds which show activity against Candida Albicans and other common pathogenic fungi (Duke, 1997).

Studies show Pau D'Arco is effective against liver cancer. In a recent study, scientists reported beta-lapachone had anti-inflammatory and anti-cancer activities in human liver cancer cells, by inhibiting their progression and metastasis (Kim, Kwon, Jeong, Kim, Kim, Choi, 2007).

Another study shows Pau D'Arco has chemopreventive properties, causing colon cancer cells to die. Active properties induce apoptosis, the process whereby a cell is destroyed (Choi, Choeng, Choi, 2003).

Warnings:
In *large* amounts, Pau D'Arco can inhibit blood clotting. Consult a physician if you have heart disease, use blood thinners, or anticoagulants.

Pregnant and nursing women should never consume Pau D'Arco because of it's toxic quinones and abortifacient properties.

Prickly Ash

Other Names: Zanthoxylum americanum (Northern), Zanthoxylum clavaherculis (Southern), Toothache Tree, Hercules Club

Parts Used: Bark and berries

Properties: Analgesic (pain relieving), alterative (deep cleansing), anti-inflammatory, anti-tumor, anti-diarrheal, antipyretic (reduces fever), anti-rheumatic, candidicide, carminative (prevents and relieves formation of gas in intestinal tract), diaphoretic (increases perspiration), emmenagogue (promotes menstruation), rubefacient (increases blood flow to the skin, causing redness), stimulant.

Indications: Toothache, sluggish circulation, arthritis, rheumatism.

PRICKLY ASH BARK

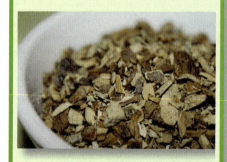

Dried chopped bark

In *The Complete Medicinal Herbal*, Penelope Ody recommends Prickly Ash Bark as a "general circulatory stimulant, promotes sweating; warming for all 'cold' conditions." She suggests a decoction of 15 g of herb in 600 ml of water (Ody, 1993).

Prickly Ash is a common tree that grows throughout Quebec, Ontario and the eastern United States as far south as Florida.

You will be able to identify this bark by it's characteristic effect on your tongue and taste buds. Chew on a tiny piece of Prickly Ash bark for a few minutes and your taste buds become so incredibly sensitive, you can taste the salt in your own saliva. The compounds in the bark send thousands of tiny prickles, numbing the area it is held against.

Also known as the Toothache Tree, Prickly Ash can be chewed or rubbed on your gums to relieve a toothache. Various native tribes from North and South America, chewed or grated the bark and left the numbing wad of bark against the aching tooth to relieve pain (Vogel, 1970).

This herb stimulates blood and lymphatic circulation, clearing acid accumulation in joints, and removing impurities from blood and tissues. In *American Indian Medicine*, Virgil J. Vogel writes that Prickly Ash was used by the Indians for medicinal qualities that 'radically remove all impurities of the blood' (Vogel, 1970).

It is energizing and warming, which makes it useful for arthritic and rheumatic conditions. Similar to the action of capsaicin, the pain reliever extracted from hot peppers; rubbing Prickly Ash into aching joints can relieve pain. Mix 1 tablespoon of ground Prickly Ash bark to 4 tablespoons of olive oil. Rub the mixture into a sore joint, wrap with a strip of cheesecloth, then a tensor bandage to hold in place and leave for as long as possible (Griggs, 1994).

Pokeweed

Other Names: Phytolacca americana L., Phytolacca decandra, Pokeweed, Coakum, Pigeonberry.

Parts Used: Dried root.

Properties: Alterative (deep cleanser), antibacterial, anti-rheumatic, anti-inflammatory, anti-cancer, anti-leukemic, anti-tumor, anti-viral, cancer-preventive, cathartic (produces bowel movements), emetic (induces vomiting in large doses), hepato-protective, immunostimulant, purgative (produces bowel movements).

Indications: Arthritis, Respiratory tract infections, laryngitis, lymphatic congestion, mumps, rheumatism, swollen lymph glands, tonsillitis, sluggish circulation, cramps in the legs, chilblains (red, itchy, inflammation in hands or feet from exposure to cold), varicose veins and varicose ulcers (Hoffman, 1996).

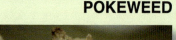

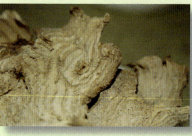

Simmer 1 teaspoon of powdered or chopped, dried root in 1 cup of water.

Take one mouthful of tea, several times throughout the day for blood and lymphatic purification, swollen glands, arthritis and rheumatism.

Be careful with Poke – See Warnings

Poke arrives early in the spring garden; by mid summer this beautiful plant grows to five feet tall, with exotic, waxy flowers, and deep purple berries.

Virgil Vogel writes in *American Indian Medicine* that Poke root was used as an antibacterial, antiviral and anti-inflammatory medicine by natives. It was also used by herbalists for its positive effects on the glands, and was prescribed for swollen or inflamed glands, breast cysts and tumors (Vogel, 1970).

Poke root affects the lungs, spleen and kidneys and has been used to treat rheumatism, arthritis and respiratory infections. Poke root is best known by its stimulating action on the lymphatic system. It is used as a lymphatic cleanser, for swollen glands, fever, tonsillitis, and mastitis in cows (Mabey, 1988).

Early Americans used the powdered root as a poultice for inflamed cow's udders (Vogel, 1970).

Dried, powdered pokeweed is used for skin infections, fungal infections, scabies, ringworm, ulcers, hemorrhoids and inflamed joints (Ody, 1993).

To support lymphatic drainage, in *The Complete Illustrated Holistic Herbal,* David Hoffman suggests, "2 parts Echinacea, 1 part Cleavers, 1 part Golden Seal, 1 part Poke root. Simmer 1 teaspoon of herb in 1 cup of water for 10 minutes. Drink three times per day" (Hoffman, 1996).

In *American Indian Medicine,* Virgil Vogel tells the story of Cadwallader Colden, a physician, botanist and statesman, who served as Lieutenant Governor of colonial New York. Apparently, Colden was told by the Mohawks to chew the root of Poke when he felt faint during travel from not eating. According to reports that Colden received, Indian Poke root was also used to cure cancer (Vogel, 1970).

FRESH DUG POKEWEED ROOT

Freshly dug fall roots from second year growth

Grind a little powder off the root and sprinkle the *dust* on skin infections, including yeast infections, athlete's foot, dry eczema, psoriasis, and scabies.

The beautiful waxy Poke flower below

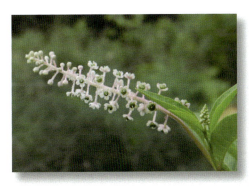

Warnings:
Fatalities have been reported in young children from garden plants. Avoid in pregnancy, it can cause fetal abnormalities. In *large* doses Pokeweed root is a violent emetic (causes vomiting) and purgative (causes bowel movements). Do not exceed recommended doses. Some people show a sensitivity to Poke. Pay close attention to gastrointestinal symptoms, when using this herb and discontinue use, if irritation results. Dried Poke root generally does not exhibit problems when used in small quantities, in combination with other supporting herbs (Tierra, 1998).

Red Clover

Other Names: Trifolium pratense L.; Fabaceae, Meadow Clover, Purple Clover, Trefoil.

Parts Used: Dried flowers, Sprouts.

Properties: Anticoagulant (reduces blood clotting), anti-angiogenic (reduces blood vessel growth to tumors), antispasmodic, astringent, calming, cancer preventive, anti-tumor, depurative (purifies blood and lymph fluids), expectorant, fungicidal, nematicidal, anti-inflammatory, immunostimulant, sedative, diuretic, deobstruent, emmenagogue, pro-estrogenic, expectorant (promotes clearance of mucous from respiratory tract), and mucolytic (reduces thickness of sputum or mucous, liquifies).

Indications: Abscesses, cancer, colds, coughs, cysts, infections with fever, infectious wounds, toxic or impure blood or lymph, cystitis and kidney infections, eczema, glandular imbalance (hormone), mucous congestion, psoriasis, skin diseases, tumors.

DRIED RED CLOVER FLOWER HEADS

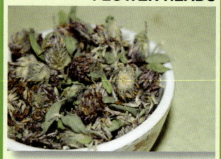

Gathered and dried throughout summer

Red clover has been used for many years to fight cancer, and is found in numerous natural herbal blends for this purpose, including Harry Hoxsey's original blend. Red clover contains hundreds of natural chemicals that include properties such as anti-cancer, anti-tumor, nematicides, fungicides, bacteriacides, immunostimulants, anti-inflammatories, and even natural sunscreens.

Search chemicals and activities *in Red Clover in* James Duke's *Phytochemical and Ethnobotanical Database.* Type in *Red Clover,* check the radio button for *Print activities with chemicals* and click *Submit Query. Here: http://www.ars-grin.gov/duke/*

Red Clover is a small plant, eight to twelve inches high, with pretty pink flowers, through summer and autumn. Gather the fresh flower heads throughout summer, as they open. Dry on screens in the shade or on tea towels in the house and pack in glass jars when completely dry. Store in a dark, cool place.

Red Clover has many beneficial properties, so many that it would be impossible to list them all here.

It is rich in calcium, phosphorus and several other minerals, which makes it strengthening for bones and teeth, and alkalizing for tissues and blood. Red Clover's demulcent, or softening and soothing properties make the tea an excellent remedy for acid indigestion (Griggs, 1994).

It is helpful in asthma, whooping cough, bronchitis and other respiratory diseases where mucous congestion is present. It soothes skin irritations like eczema, psoriasis, acne and boils, and protects the skin against sun damage. Red Clover contains coumarins which help to gently thin the blood (Reader's Digest, 1998).

Red Clover is also high in hormone balancing phytoestrogens and has been used to relieve the uncomfortable symptoms of PMS and menopause.

It's most noble quality is that of purifying the blood, where Red Clover is one of the best alteratives, alongside Burdock. Blood purifiers gently remove toxins and excess moisture and stimulate the immune system's production of white blood cells. Alteratives have been used for centuries in cancer therapy to cleanse the blood and balance the fluids of the body.

GROWING RED CLOVER

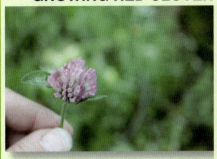

Sweet, organic Red Clover flower

Red Clover is very easy to grow in your garden. Purchase Red Clover seeds from a farm supply store or garden center. I used sprouting seeds from the health food store, and threw them into one end of the vegetable garden. Now there is a flourishing community of pretty Red Clover flower heads for anti-cancer and hormone balancing tea all winter. They are simple to dry too, just leave them on a cotton tea towel, underneath a ceiling fan if possible, out of direct sun.

Toss the fresh flowers into a salad of baby greens, with thin slivers of French shallot and slivered almonds. They add a delicate, sweet flavor, chopped or whole. Serve with a slightly sweet vinaigrette, blended white wine vinegar, sunflower oil, and a small dollop of unpasteurized liquid honey. Add chopped fresh tarragon leaves.

Red Clover flowers contain genistein, a chemical with anti-angiogenic properties, useful in reducing the growth of blood vessels to tumors (Duke, 1997).

114

My mother's tumor was small and round, with a hole in the middle where a blood vessel was attached. Tumors require a constant supply of sugar and as they grow and mature, they release biochemical signals which promote the growth of blood vessels into themselves. This process is called Angiogenesis.

Soon we will talk about many other plants and their foods, who inherently carry these anti-angiogenic properties.

A search for Red Clover on the University of Michigan-Dearborn, *Native American Ethonobotany database*, returns the following traditional remedies, using Red Clover for cancer. Here: http://herb.umd.umich.edu/

- Shinnecock Drug is used in Cancer treatment. A teaspoon of powdered flower is mixed in boiling water and drank (University of Michigan-Dearborn, 2010).

- Thompson Drug (Cancer Treatment) Infusion of heads taken for stomach cancer (University of Michigan-Dearborn, 2010).

RED CLOVER TEA

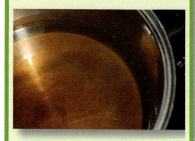

Large Pot of Red Clover Tea

Red clover tea has a pleasant taste, delicate and slightly sweet, and may be taken once or twice a day for medicinal purposes. Use 2 teaspoons of dried crushed petals, or 6 fresh or dried flower heads. Pour boiling water over herbs and steep 10 minutes or more.

Red Clover flowers make a refreshing iced tea. Make a large pot of tea (like above) and refrigerate until cool. Add fresh squeezed lemon juice and a sweetener (stevia, raw unpasteurized honey or raw agave syrup) to taste. Serve with a wedge of lemon.

Red Clover is a marvelous blood depurative and formidable remedy for leprosy, pellagra and malignant tumors.

Jethro Kloss, Back to Eden, 1971.

Rhubarb

Other Names: Rheum palmatum, Rheum rhabarbarum L., Rheum officinale, Rheum rhaponticum, Chinese Rhubarb, Da Huang, Turkey Rhubarb, Wild Rhubarb.

Parts Used: Rhizome.

Properties: Anti-Cancer, anti-tumor, anti-mutagenic, alterative (deep cleanser), antibiotic, astringent, anthelmintic (destroys parasitic worms), cathartic (produces bowel movements), immunostimulant, laxative, purgative (produces bowel movements), vulnerary (heals wounds).

Indications: The Chinese name for Rhubarb, *Ta huang*, means great yellow, referring to it's large medicinal rhizome (Reader's Digest, 1998).

There are many varieties of Rhubarb. Rene Caisse's recipe called for Turkey Rhubarb root, which is readily available. Garden Rhubarb root can be substituted, but has less potent properties. Avoid the leaves of Rhubarb plants as they can be poisonous, even fatal.

RHUBARB LEMONADE

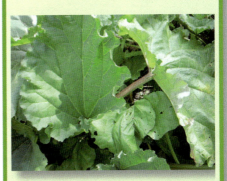

Poisonous Leaves, edible stalks and medicinal rhizome.

Rhubarb stalks are a delicious spring treat in many countries around the world, used to make pies, jams and rhubarb sauce.

To make rhubarb lemonade, juice 3 or 4 rhubarb stalks, add the juice of one lemon, fresh water and stevia, unpasteurized liquid honey or raw agave nectar to taste. A sweet, tart and refreshing summer drink.

RHUBARB ROOT TEA

Rhubarb root can be made into a tea. Pour water just off the boil over a teaspoon of dried, powdered root, let steep for 5 to 10 minutes. Drink up!

Rhubarb root is a bit unusual, in that it provides therapeutic healing in small quantities through it's astringent action, but is a strong laxative when used in larger quantities. It has been used to treat both diarrhea and constipation (Reader's Digest, 1998).

A study by Qing Huang et al. in 2007, 'Anti-cancer properties of anthraquinones from rhubarb,' showed Rhubarb to have valuable anti-cancer properties that inhibited cellular proliferation, induced apoptosis or programmed cell death, prevented metastasis, and contained aloe-emodin, a powerful chemical with anti-tumor properties. Huang concludes that Rhubarb has promising anti-cancer properties with broad therapeutic potential in treating cancer (Huang, 2007).

The phytochemical Emodin is listed under Rhubarb in James Duke's *Phytochemical and Ethnobotanical Database.* The biological activities listed for this phytochemical include: antibacterial, anti-leukemic, anti-lymphomic, anti-mutagenic, antineoplastic, anti-sarcomic, anti-tumor (breast) and anti-viral (Dr. Duke's *Phytochemical and Ethnobotanical Database,* 1998). Here: http:// www.ars-grin.gov/duke/ plants.html.

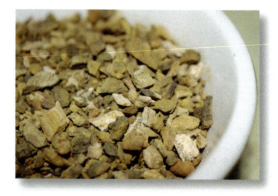

Dried Turkey Rhubarb Root

Warnings:

The *fresh leaves* of several rhubarb species contain toxic oxalates, and can cause burning pain, vomiting, liver and kidney damage and are potentially fatal.

Never use rhubarb root if you are pregnant or nursing, or if you have irritable bowel syndrome, diverticular disease, colitis or Crohn's disease.

Rhubarb root should not be used for an extended period of time.

Slippery Elm

Other Names: Ulmus rubra, Ulmus fulva, Indian Elm, Sweet Elm, Moose Elm, Red Elm.

Parts Used: Dried inner bark.

Properties: Anti-Cancer, anti-leukemic, anti-nausea, anti-tumor, astringent, calming, demulcent (soothes and softens), emollient (softens and smoothes, immunostimulant, laxative, nutritive, soothing lubricant, vulnerary (heals wounds).

Indications: Bruises, cancer, gastrointestinal ulcers and inflammation, sore or dry throat, tightness in chest, weakened conditions, wounds.

Slippery Elm inner bark contains large amounts of mucilage, the gelatinous polysaccharide, or slippery substance you feel when water is added to the soft bark. Rub a tiny bit of bark and water between your fingers and you can *feeeel* how this substance soothes inflammation.

Richard Mabey in *The New Age Herbalist*, recommends the inner bark as a soothing remedy for inflammation in the gastro-intestinal tract. It soothes, lubricates and checks diarrhea with its mildly astringent action (Mabey, 1988).

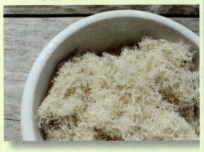

SLIPPERY ELM BARK

Dried inner bark

David Hoffman recommends a decoction made from Slippery Elm bark for gastritis, gastric or duodenal ulcers, enteritis and colitis.

In *The Complete Illustrated Holistic Herbal*, Hoffman suggests using 1 part of powdered bark to 8 parts of water. The mixture is simmered gently for ten or fifteen minutes. The dose is half a cup, three times a day.

Slippery Elm can be used as a poultice for boils, abscesses or ulcers. Make a poultice for wounds by mixing powdered Slippery Elm bark with enough water to form a paste. Apply to wound, cover with a clean bandage, and replace as needed (Hoffman, 1996).

118

Michael Tierra, in *The Way Of Herbs*, suggests using a tea of powdered Slippery Elm bark and honey to soothe sore and irritated throats, coughs, and dryness of the throat and lungs (Tierra, 1998).

Slippery Elm bark Lozenges are available in health food stores, pharmacies and some grocery stores.

Both Tierra and Mabey report the use of slippery elm bark as a nutritious food for debilitated patients.

Tierra suggests using ginseng tea to prepare a gruel for severely debilitated patients. Buy Ginseng tea bags or pour boiling water over powdered Ginseng root and steep for ten minutes (Tierra, 1998).

In *American Indian Medicine*, Vogel tells how, "Samuel Stearns, (who wrote the first book on American herbs in 1801, the classic American Herbal – Materia Medica), referred to Slippery Elm bark as good in chronic, cutaneous eruptions, in suppression of urine, dropsy, inflammation and hard tumors" (Vogel, 1970).

SLIPPERY ELM GRUEL

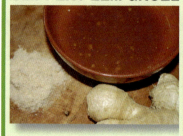

This gruel is similar to the decoction in the previous green box, for gastritis and ulcers, but is made with much less water, so is of thicker consistency, more like a porridge.

Simmer powdered Slippery Elm Bark in enough water to make a thick, creamy porridge. This gruel was made with a teaspoon of unpasteurized liquid honey, and a good pinch each of dried cinnamon, ginger and a smaller pinch of nutmeg.

It is soothing, nourishing, very delicious and is taken easily by infants and sick people.

Potassium Iodide

Properties: Expectorant, iodine source, potassium source.

The expectorant activity of Potassium Iodide promotes clearance of mucus from the respiratory tract.

I believe, this ingredient added to Bitter Tonic Tea, helped my mother cough out tumors from her lung and bronchi tubes. The formula seems to have more expectorant qualities when I add Potassium Iodide, as I have made it without this ingredient many times also. Every so often, during the time she was taking the tea, she would enter into a coughing fit for two or three days, and it would end when she coughed out a small tumor. Then she seemed fine for another few weeks, until it would happen again.

The entry in *Taber's Cyclopedic Medical Dictionary* states, "Potassium iodide KI; colorless or white crystals having a faint odor of iodine, used as an expectorant. Potassium Iodide is recommended for use following exposure to radioactive iodides downwind from a nuclear reactor accident. The rationale is that it blocks the uptake of radioactive iodides by the thyroid gland, thus preventing or decreasing the chance of developing cancer of the thyroid many years later" (Venes, 2001).

Consider the method of testing for thyroid cancer in people. First we are told to drink from a small glass, which holds a liquid impregnated with radioactive Iodine. This radioactive Iodine is taken up by our thyroid gland. Now when the radiologist scans our thyroid, he can see it on the scan, because it is glowing with radioactive Iodine.

Does this sound safe to you?

Radioactive Iodine causes thyroid cancer and dietary Iodine protects against it.

Now that you know the truth, would you still drink thyroid-cancer causing, radioactive Iodine, just so doctors can *see* if you have thyroid cancer?

What if you *did not* have thyroid cancer, and just exposed your thyroid gland to radioactive Iodine?

An enlarged thyroid gland is often due to a deficiency of Iodine, a main cause of goiter. Goiter is defined as, "Thyroid gland enlargement. An enlarged thyroid gland may be caused by thyroiditis, benign thyroid nodules, malignancy, iodine deficiency, or any condition that causes hyperfunction or hypofunction of the gland" (Venes, 2001).

It would make sense to test for a nutritional deficiency before anything else because it is so easy to reverse . . . and so common!

I am certain that if you *did* have thyroid cancer, you probably would not want to damage more of your thyroid cells and increase your risk for more cancer, by drinking radioactive Iodine.

Would you?

POTASSIUM IODIDE PROTECTS THYROID FROM RADIOACTIVE IODINE [131]I

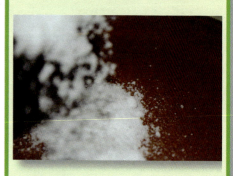

Potassium Iodide supplementation can be used to protect the Thyroid gland in case of exposure to radioactive Iodine ^{131}I from nuclear accident and medical x-rays. Improve your Iodine intake by eating Iodine rich sea vegetables like Nori, Wakame, Kombu, Chlorella and Kelp. Some sea salts have trace amounts of Iodine, check the label.

The study, 'Risk of Thyroid Cancer After Exposure to Iodine ^{131}I in Childhood,' shows how the use of potassium iodide protected the thyroid gland and reduced the risk of thyroid cancer in children exposed to radioactive Iodine ^{131}I, after the Chernobyl nuclear accident. The study concludes, iodine supplementation in deficient populations may *substantially* reduce risk of thyroid cancer caused by exposure to radioactive iodines from medical diagnostic and therapeutic procedures as well as radiative accidents such as Chernobyl (Cardis, Kesminiene, Ivanov, Malakhova, Shibata, Khrouch, et al., 2005).

33 Bitter Tonic Tea™ ~ The Recipe

Properties: Anti-cancer, Anti-tumor, Anti-candida, Anti-fungal, Detoxifying, Cleansing, Nutritionally Supportive, Expectorant, Metabolism Boosting, Immuno-stimulant, Laxative, Anticatarrhal (reduces catarrh, inflammation of nose and air passages), Antigoitrogenic (reduces goiter, supports thyroid), and many, many more (see individual herbs).

This tea is rich in cancer fighting phytochemicals, antioxidants, vitamins and minerals and provides a rich source of potent anti-cancer properties.

This recipe is simple enough to make the tea yourself in your own kitchen. Herbal teas similar to this one, have been used for centuries, and are still used by people all over the world.

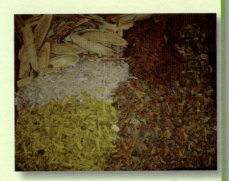

BITTER TONIC TEA HERBS

Dried herbs from Herbalist

These herbs have been used to heal cancer for centuries and are widely available. Some are even considered foods in many countries. For example, Burdock root is a staple food in Japan and Red Clover is used as rich fodder for farm animals, and as a hormone balancing tea for women all over the world.

This combination of herbs cleanses your organs, tissues and blood, kills pathogenic organisms, including fungus, all while gently supporting and rebuilding your body and it's billions of cells.

The formula uses some of the same powerful herbs as the famous early cancer teas. It is similar in effect to Hoxsey's formula which was used by Hoxsey himself from the early 1900s to the 1950s, and by many practitioners today; and Rene Caisse's formula, Essiac™, which is easy to duplicate, or buy from most health food stores, under the name of Flor-Essence™, made by Flora (Flora Essence, 2010).

The company does not sell its products online, so you must go to a health food store. Their herbal blend includes some of the same herbs as other well known formulas; Burdock root, Sheep Sorrel leaves, Slippery Elm bark, Watercress, Turkish Rhubarb root, Kelp, Blessed Thistle, and Red Clover flowers (Flora Essence, 2010).

Hoxsey's formula is of particular interest. Claims say his formula has healed thousands from many different types of cancer, including lung, uterine, breast cancers and melanoma. Many of his claims have been proven in U.S. courts during cases brought against him by U.S. medical officials from the FDA and the American Medical Association, during the early to mid-1900s.

My version of the formula has been tested on many types of growth, including melanoma and metastasized bowel cancer, with astounding results. In most cases, healing was visible within days, and regression of growths took anywhere from two weeks to three months.

In the case of my mother's metastasized bowel cancer in her lung, while drinking the tea off and on for several months, it caused expulsion of small pea-like tumors, that were coughed out of her lung (See Histopathology Report from Laboratory that analyzed the tumor, on page 33).

Most health food stores carry these herbs, or you can search out a master herbalist, which may require going to a city if you live in a rural area. Some herbs can be ethically harvested in the wild or grown in your own garden. See entries for individual herbs.

EASY BITTER TONIC TEA

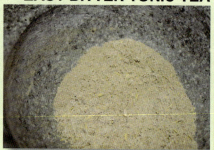

Although this version is not quite as strong as the one above, it is very simple and quick to make. Measure all the herbs from the original recipe below, into a glass bowl and stir together. Don't forget the red clover flowers. Store the bulk of your herbal mixture in a large glass jar, in a cool, dark place. Store the mixture for immediate use on your counter.

Grind 2 tablespoons of herbal mixture in a mortar and pestle till well broken up. I always throw in a few more red clover flowers, because of their potent anti-cancer properties . . . Put them in a two cup, loose leaf teapot and pour over water just off the boil. Put the lid on tightly and let steep for a good twenty minutes. Drink one cup and leave the other to steep longer, all day if you want. Put it in the refrigerator after it has cooled.

You can apply this tea topically too. Just soak a cotton ball in the tea, tape it on and see what happens . . . ☺

If you are worried about the ingredients, take a list to your doctor. If SHe truly wants to help you, SHe will not discourage you.

There is nothing in the tea that is harmful in the *quantities* given, but please take note of the warnings on the individual herbs, as well as the warnings at the bottom of this recipe. Herbs have powerful properties and it is important to respect this.

Step 1 ~ Simmer Roots, Stems and Bark:

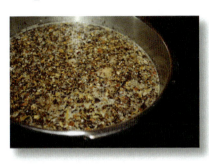

☹ = These Herbs Carry Warnings! Buy chopped, dried herbs. The smaller the chop the better, which helps to increase the surface area, and extraction rate of medicinal properties.

Simmer barks and roots in fresh water in a large crockpot, on low for one hour; or place the herbs in a large pressure cooker or pot with a tight lid. Bring to boil (without the lid), turn down heat and simmer for 20 minutes. Take off heat, seal lid and let steep for 30 minutes.

Always simmer bark, stems and roots to extract their properties. Pour boiling water over flowers and leaves to steep, to protect their more delicate qualities.

Burdock root	*2 cups*
Pau D'Arco bark	*1 cup* ☹
Slippery Elm bark	*1/2 cup*
Licorice root	*1/2 cup* ☹
Cascara Sagrada bark	*1/2 cup* ☹
Berberis root	*1/2 cup* ☹
Prickly Ash bark	*1/4 cup*
Poke root	*1/4 cup* ☹
Turkey Rhubarb root	*1/2 cup* ☹

Step 2 ~ Prepare bottles
When tea is almost finished, wash glass jars and lids in hot soapy water. Rinse well and cover with fresh, cold water in large canning pot. Bring to boil and boil hard for 5-6 minutes.

Step 3 ~ Steep Leaves and Flowers
Boil a full kettle of water, pour over flowers and let steep.
Red Clover flowers	*4 cups*

Step 4 ~ Add Potassium Iodide

Add potassium iodide salts to the red clover tea and stir until dissolved.

Potassium Iodide   *2 tablespoons*

Step 5 ~ Strain and bottle tea

Strain both teas through cheesecloth or a fine strainer, pressing gently. Combine the teas and put back on the stove in a large pot. Bring the temperature back up to boiling point for 2 or 3 minutes. Lower heat. Keep it hot (not boiling) while you fill the jars. Lift hot bottles out of the water one at a time, fill with hot tea, put on lid, and put back in boiling water. Remove some water or your pot will overflow. Boil for 3-5 minutes, maximum. This will kill anything that may have entered the tea during bottling. Remove the bottles from the pot and sit on a tea towel until cool. Do not let the bottles touch. Never tighten your seals after removing from the water, as this may cause them to unseal. Please know what you are doing when canning hot liquids, as this can be dangerous.

Refrigerate the tea when cooled completely. The tea will last up to six months refrigerated, not opened. Once open, use the tea within three to four weeks. Never put a spoon or other utensil in the tea. Shake, then pour it onto a teaspoon. Recap immediately, and put back in the refrigerator.

Dose:

Start with 1 teaspoon morning and 1 teaspoon evening. Work up to 1 tablespoon morning and 1 tablespoon evening.

This tea is strongly detoxifying. Go slow at first. If your bowels move too quickly then take less and slowly work up to the maximum amount. You can tweak the formula to have less laxative herbs like Cascara Sagrada, Poke root and Rhubarb root.

All the herbs are considered very safe and effective, in the quantities here. If you have questions about the ingredients, please research them further, or consult a qualified master herbalist or natural practitioner.

To explain the strength of the medicine you are about to make, I will tell you a funny story.

My husband Bob was just getting over a cold, when he started to get worse, not better. He started hacking and coughing constantly. This went on for four or five days, when we realized he was clearly having problems. The children and I started to think there was something terribly wrong.

That morning, I opened the refrigerator, and noticed that almost the whole bottle of Bitter Tonic Tea was gone. I had only made it the week before, so it could not possibly be gone already! I looked at the bottle, with a puzzled look on my face, shut the door to the refrigerator, turned to my daughter and asked, "Who drank all this tea?"

"Probably Dad. I saw him swigging out of it this morning," she replied, turning down the corners of her mouth sarcastically.

I walked to the living room and asked my husband, "Have you been drinking any Bitter Tonic Tea lately?"

"Yes," he coughed out. "I've been taking it for the last few days. Why?"

"How much have you been taking?," I asked him, while at the same time realizing why his body had been purging so intensely.

He admitted he was taking large swigs of tea, twice a day. The directions above say start with one teaspoon twice a day. In five days he had taken over two cups of tea! As soon as he backed off and took the proper dose, the cleansing slowed down and he began to feel better, his coughing, hacking and purging stopped and he was back to his regular old self, except now he was without a cold!

He uses the tea if he gets a cold or respiratory infection, along with fresh garlic or garlic pills, to stop the infection short and cure it before it gets hold of him. He swears by this method.

The moral of the story is:

Follow the directions, this is strong medicine!

Warnings:
If you are on medications, there can be risks that some herbs cause medications to have a stronger effect. Be careful. Herbs carry desirable properties naturally, such as blood thinning, lowering blood pressure and lowering blood sugar levels. Medications combined with herbs can cause amplified effects. Consult an expert master herbalist, physician or other qualified practitioner to be sure this formula will not interact with medications you may be taking.

Notes:

If any of the herbs are not available to you, do not despair, make the tea anyway. All the herbs have multiple anti-cancer and antifungal properties. They work best to combat cancer together but also work well alone.

If your pharmacist will not sell you potassium iodide, try a different pharmacy, and if you cannot get it, do not worry, the tea will still work!

Potassium Iodide acts as an expectorant, cleans your respiratory system, boosts your metabolism by providing iodine for your thyroid gland and potassium for the function and fluid balance of all your cells.

Eat lots of fresh, raw fruits and vegetables for Potassium.

Our richest source of Iodine comes from sea vegetables.

34 Our Incredible Bodies

Our bodies are an amazing mixture of energy and biological matter. They always strive to heal . . . always. Think of how quickly your skin seals and repairs itself after a wound. Think of a bruise, first red and hot with inflammation. Constant healing takes place as the bruise turns from purple to yellow and then disappears. A body miraculously heals after a broken leg or a surgically removed kidney. Predictable, continuous repair. Amazing isn't it?

Just as amazing, incredible and true is the fact that our bodies heal from cancer, in exactly the same way.

Why then, do we as a modern, intelligent society, hinder the healing process with poisonous chemotherapeutic drugs, cancer inducing radiation therapy and mutilating, surgical removal of body parts?

Why do we allow our bodies to be so debilitated and harmed?

Why do we continue to use procedures that are clearly not working?

Your body has built in resistance to cancer, and uses the nutrients and chemicals obtained from food to protect itself against damage caused by mutagenic poisons, excessive heat or cold, radiation, pathogenic organisms and toxins produced during normal metabolic processes.

For example, your skin naturally carries a protective layer of the antioxidant, vitamin C. Close to the equator, where the sun is strongest, you find the highest concentration of vitamin C rich foods. High levels of vitamin C are known to protect your body against cancers of all kinds, including skin cancer. Andrew Saul reports, in 'Topical Vitamin C Stops Basal Cell Carcinoma', that vitamin C has been used topically against basal cell carcinoma with much success (Saul, 2007).

Phytoestrogens contained in many natural foods, the antioxidant Indole 3 carbinol and the sulforaphanes from cruciferous vegetables, like broccoli, cabbage, brussel sprouts, cauliflower and kale, protect our reproductive tissues from excess growth stimulation by estrogen. Estrogen of course, is a natural hormone essential to your body, but the use of synthetic estrogens has been implicated in reproductive cancers in both men and women, and conversely, the use of natural phytoestrogens from plants, are reported to have a protective and beneficial effect against reproductive cancers.

Under normal circumstances your immune system is extremely adept at handling the destruction of damaged and cancerous cells, but if you continue to expose your cells to mutagenic substances and do not provide your tissues with the nutrients needed to protect themselves and repair damage to their DNA and other structures, tumors arise, and cancer can flourish.

In New York, teams are finding that young patients with a precancerous condition of the larynx called laryngeal papilloma, which normally requires repeated operations to remove small growths on the voice box, don't need surgery after drinking enriched cabbage juice . . . At Pittsburgh, Chivendra Singh and Sanja Srivastava have extinguished cancer in cell cultures grown from cancerous ovaries and the prostate by giving them concentrated chemicals taken from these same vegetables (cabbage like vegetables called cruciferae).

Devra Davis, 2007.

Cytotoxic lymphocytes, known as Natural Killer Cells, circulate throughout your body's fluids, and are in highest concentrations within your lymph fluid and lymph nodes. NK cells recognize chemicals on the surface of cells which identify them as invaders or mutated cells. They attack the target cell by releasing chemicals into it's membrane, disintegrating first the membrane, then the core nucleus of the cancer cell (Marieb, 2003).

As the cell is destroyed, wastes are carried away by macrophages, and the tumor disintegrates, as if it never existed!

What a beautiful thing! The key to curing cancer is to *promote* and *accelerate* the healing process, which is already taking place within your body. How do you do that? Just follow the **10 Key Principles of Healing** . . .

35   10 Key Principles of Healing

These principles can be applied to almost any illness as they provide universal benefits by cleansing and rebuilding your body, protecting your trillions of cells, supporting your fluids, tissues, organs and systems, and promoting optimum functioning of your immunity with a fully functioning lymphatic system and a fortress of disease fighting cells.

These principles work *with* your body, not against it.

The first principle is;

1.   Use Your Power!
Use Your Power by having a proactive approach to healing. Just thinking about healing is not enough, but it's a start! You must take action and heal yourself. No one can do this for you. Visualize yourself already healed, the way you want to be. You will begin to build a foundation of strength to cure yourself, and most importantly, you will learn to trust your inner guidance. This principle is so important, some people have effectively used it as the only tool to cure cancer and other illnesses.

2.   Cleanse and Detoxify!
The next step is to clean the years of accumulated acids, wastes, toxins and pathogens from your blood, tissues and organs. You will soon learn simple ways to cleanse and detoxify your body.

3.   Super Nutrition!
Eating the right foods is paramount to the healing process. Without adequate nutrition, no organism can realize the *serenity* that comes with good health. Withdraw nutrition from any organism alive; plant, animal or otherwise, and they will wither and die. There are many foods that offer the benefits of *super nutrition*. I'll cover them in detail soon.

4.   Befriend Herbs!
Although the knowledge of herbs and their properties has been known for centuries, a stigma surrounds the use of them. People think that herbal medicine formulas are secret and only special, knowledgeable people can make them. This could not be further from the truth. Armed with basic

knowledge about herbs, every person with a kitchen and simple tools can make effective anti-cancer medicines.

5. Get Rid Of The Acid!

It is imperative to create an environment where cancer cannot live and flourish by balancing your pH. With a test you can perform at home in seconds, and simple diet changes, you will learn how to check and control your pH. You will learn what to eat to increase the alkalinity of your blood and tissues and decrease acid accumulation. Proper pH balance limits the colonization and proliferation of pathogens like viruses, bacteria and fungi, including Candida Albicans; most notably known for causing yeast infections; least notably known for being a main part of the cancerous process.

6. Natural Supplementation!

Natural supplementation has been going on forever. Why pay for expensive supplements when foods do the same thing? One of the most valuable things you will learn, is to supplement your diet with nutrient rich super foods that nourish and protect your body. You will find details about which foods they are, how to slip them into your diet, and how to prepare them to get maximum, natural supplementation.

7. Move and Breathe!

Some people are afraid of *exercise*, but it does not have to be that way. Exercise can be fun when you do what you enjoy. Playing sports can be strenuous but some people love the exercise that comes with going after the ball. Yoga is an addictive practice that some people cannot get enough of, once they find a great teacher. Walking can be done anywhere, by just about anyone, with only a pair of shoes. Even gardening or stretching, or touching your toes are all exercise. Just find what you love and keep doing it. Exercise increases breathing, and breathing deeply is one of the most important tools against cancer. More about this soon.

8. Sunshine and Vitamin D!

Good ole sunshine. The news just keeps getting better. Yes, you should soak up the sun. Book that trip to the beach now – just do it! Then throw out your expensive sunscreens and find out what you have been missing by listening to fear mongering.

9. Be Good To Yourself!

Relieve stress, have fun, laugh, meditate, sleep! Just relax! Are you tired? Do you feel guilty about taking time for yourself? Stop it! You need lots of rest, relaxation, fun and sleep, free from stress to heal your body. Sounds good, doesn't it?

10. Avoid The Causes And . . . No, Everything Does Not Cause Cancer!

This principle could not be any more obvious. There are plenty of things we are exposing ourselves to every day that cause cancer. Become knowledgeable about what you put in or on your body. Denial about chemicals and toxins will not keep you safe, education will.

These principles will cause you to feel great and look great. You get to keep your body parts and your hair and nails will never fall out!

Read on, because the next chapter begins to uncover the ten key principles in detail.

36   Principle 1 ~ Use Your Power!

Use *your power* to be proactive, take action and be responsible for your health, instead of relying on fate or allowing others to make *your* decisions.

Your body heals from cancer, the same way it heals from a cut or a bruise. Your body always strives to heal.

Believe it! If you do not believe it and just keep telling yourself you will heal, that is not enough. You have to really know it and take actions on the knowledge that it is possible to cure yourself of any ailment.

Which actions?

They will reveal themselves throughout the 10 Key Principles of Healing.

Remove Your Fear
Do *not* buy into the fear of cancer.

Stay in control of your emotions and do not let what others say upset you.

Many others have been told they had only a few weeks to live, but they walked away and never looked back. Those same brave people are still very alive and well many years after being told they would die.

Everyone has their own opinions and reasons for promoting a certain therapy or treatment. You must step back to acknowledge and observe any biases that exist *before* you make *any* decisions.

If you still have questions after reading this book, look in the resource section as there are many reliable and unbiased resources, studies, articles, databases and informative websites listed there for your future reference and study.

Fear is proven to suppress your immune system, hampering its ability to perform the most important job of producing natural killer cells that actively seek out and destroy cancer cells. Do not let fear have control over your health and your ability to fight cancer.

Dr. Bruce Lipton reminds us in *Biology Of Belief*, that we can choose the filter through which we view our world.

You can filter your life with rose-colored beliefs that will help your body grow or you can use a dark filter that turns everything black and makes your body/mind more susceptible to disease. You can live a life of fear or live a life of love. You have the choice! But I can tell you that if you choose to see a world full of love, your body will respond by growing in health. If you choose to believe that you live in a dark world full of fear, your body's health will be compromised as you physiologically close yourself down in a protection response.

Dr. Bruce Lipton, Ph. D., *The Biology Of Belief*, 2009.

Placebo Or Nocebo, It's All Mind Over Health!

We often hear about the placebo effect. This is a simulated medical intervention in the form of sugar pills, which are given to people in a study, instead of the real medication being studied. A placebo produces a positive, therapeutic effect, similar to the medication, even though the treatment is fake. In other words, the participant's health improves simply because they *believe* they are given medicine which might help them.

Opposite to the placebo effect is the nocebo effect. The nocebo effect is very real and can cause people to believe they are ill, when there is actually nothing wrong with them. An example of the nocebo effect would be a diagnosis of breast cancer in a woman who does not actually have breast cancer. This is known as a false positive. She believes what she is being told, even though it is a mistake.

This belief can cause illness to manifest, despite the fact that there is nothing actually wrong! The nocebo effect can also lead a person to accept harmful treatments like chemotherapy, increasing their risk for cancer, for a disease they do not even have!

Earlier you learned from a study that showed, after ten mammograms a woman's chance of a false positive is 49.1%! (Christiansen, Wang,

134

Barton, Kreuter, Elmore, Gelfand et al., 2000). The nocebo effect would play a large role if a woman is told she has breast cancer when she really does not.

In medicine, the nocebo effect can be as powerful as the placebo effect, a fact you should keep in mind every time you step into a doctor's office. By their words and demeanor, physicians can convey hope-deflating messages to their patients, messages that are, I believe, completely unwarranted... Another example is the potential power of the statement: "You have six months to live." If you choose to believe your doctor's message, you are not likely to have much more time on this Earth.

Dr. Bruce Lipton, Ph. D., *The Biology Of Belief*, 2009.

True Stories

Use true stories of natural healing from other people to prove to yourself that you too can heal yourself. There are powerful and motivational messages in these stories. There are some stories in this book but there are thousands of stories all around you of people who have healed from cancer and other diseases.

Visit *www.IncredibleHealingJournals.com* to see, hear and read incredible stories of natural healing.

When you have heard enough stories, and gained enough confidence then you will be able to reach out and grab the light like they did. *Trust* yourself and *know* your body's infinite healing wisdom.

Billy Best

Billy Best took matters into his own hands and refused to let his health be a product of conditions created by others. He took control, learned what he had to do and made the changes necessary. He was so proactive, he fled his home to save his life! Now he is alive and well without cancer or damage to his body from conventional treatments. Best of all, Billy has a story of incredible courage and inspiration to share with others. To learn more about Billy's story, or to support Billy by purchasing Essiac™ through his website, go to www.billybest.net. Billy started on nine ounces of Essiac™ tea daily and continued for six months. He takes three or four ounces daily to prevent recurrence (Best & Best, 2010).

Billy also made drastic changes to his diet, and like the others whose stories are in this book, Billy followed the principles of healing by avoiding red meat, dairy products, sugar and sodas. He eats fresh, organic produce, water, whole, natural unprocessed foods, and takes supplements to build his immune system. Billy's mother reports on his website that in March 1995, two and a half months after beginning these natural therapies, his cancer was gone. It has never returned (Best & Best, 2010). Only two months . . .

Linda Devine
Remember Linda Devine and how she healed herself of breast cancer? She refused inferior treatments for cancer and chose natural healing instead. She *knew* she deserved better than having her breast cut open and bombarded by radiation. She trusted her instincts when it came to her health and it paid off immensely. Now she uses this experience to teach others to be proactive and heal naturally.

Jay Kordich
Jay Kordich trusted his instincts, gained the knowledge necessary and juiced his way back to health. He took a proactive approach and healed himself of bladder cancer.

Jay, known as The Juice Daddy, at www.juicedaddy.com, has been an inspiration to the world for decades. He sent a message to share with you.

When I was 25 years old, I was a dedicated football player for USC, the Green Bay Packers, until one day, soon after signing, I pulled a muscle that made it impossible for me to play football any longer. To this day, my leg will never be the same, as there is a big tear near my thigh.

During that time, and soon after leaving football, I contracted bladder cancer, and my wife left with our two young boys who I never saw again, until I turned 70 years old.

My doctor at USC is the one who diagnosed the tumor in my bladder, as I was urinating blood for many weeks. Three weeks later, I went to New York to see Dr. Gerson, the doctor to Albert Schweitzer and went on his juicing program. Within two weeks of being on his program, I stopped urinating blood, my energy levels were sky high and I felt I was going to live again, even though my personal life was a mess, I felt I had another chance to live.

I dedicated my entire life then, at the age of 26 years old, back in 1949, to not just sell juicers, but to teach others what I did, and how I got well, and how others can be well and stay well by consuming fresh vegetable juices and by eating a vegetarian diet.

Now that I am 86, I do not have cancer, and I am vitally alive and feeling energy every day I wake up. In the year 1990, I was blessed enough to be discovered (after 42 years of working day and night) on television and was able to share what I knew and had been teaching for so many decades about the power of juicing. We reached all of America and the world with our message, selling over one billion dollars in juicer sales, and my book, the Juiceman's Power of Juicing sold close to 3 million books.

I retired in the year 2000, but now in the year 2009, I am coming out of retirement with a new juicer and a wonderful juicing and lifestyle program I spent 62 years accumulating. It's my life's work and I hope to share it with everyone who is interested in living a vital LIFE, rich with appreciation for Nature, for Living Foods and for a Gentle way of Living.

"

Jay Kordich, The Juice Daddy, 2010.

Kerri Howarth

I met Kerri several years ago, but really got to know her story through an interview about her situation. Kerri has always been healthy and very slim, but in 2002 she began to experience multiple symptoms, including headaches and depression, the most disturbing symptom was a weight gain of almost seventy pounds over only a few months.

Doctors in Canada dismissed her symptoms and could not identify the cause. It was not until Kerri travelled to the United States for an MRI, that she found out a tumor on her pituitary gland was causing hormone levels in all her glands to fluctuate in wide swings, resulting in the severe symptoms she was experiencing.

Although a doctor in Canada refused to test Kerri for a pituitary tumor, pooh-poohing her symptoms, and saying she must be eating too many muffins, doctors in the United States, in possession of Kerri's MRI wanted to operate and remove her entire pituitary gland along with the tumor, which would mean she would have to take synthetic hormones for the rest of her life.

Kerri sought refuge in her own world away from the pressures and confusion of the medical industry and decided to take control herself.

Kerri switched to a raw vegan diet, lost all the weight, and now lives a healthy and active life. To see Kerri's interview or read the transcript, visit 'Pituitary Tumor on Raw Food Diet.' Here: www.thegoodwitch.ca/pituitary/

I was going to appointments, I was feeling frustrated and I decided at some point, it's my life! Power of thought, change in diet, I went to a vegan diet then switched in a few months to a raw diet. I did a lot of research because it's personally empowering to take control of your life.

Kerri Howarth, 2008.

138

Yvonne Chamberlain

Yvonne Chamberlain was diagnosed with a deadly black melanoma on her leg, twenty-eight years ago. Doctors pronounced that she had only six weeks to live and urged her to let them take her leg off to prevent the cancer from spreading and killing her.

Yvonne did not cave to their fear mongering and dismal predictions. Instead she used common sense, walked away and chose life! In Yvonne's words, "Why would I let them amputate my leg, if I only had six weeks to live?"

Yvonne is now a living testament to the power of natural therapies for cancer; with several grandchildren, a published book, her own successful internet businesses, and both of her legs . . .

Twenty eight years ago the medical profession gave me six weeks to live after diagnosing black melanoma. They suggested wider incision after the biopsy and the possibility of taking my leg off to prevent the spread . . . it is my life mission and purpose, to make a difference to those people who have been told like I had . . . get yourself ready to die, you only have six weeks to live . . .

Yvonne Chamberlain, 2010.

Now Yvonne spends her days teaching others to heal themselves. She coaches others to be *totally healthy,* and has recorded her experience and knowledge in a book entitled, *Why Me, Kicking Cancer and Other Life Changing Stuff.*

In the following years after treating myself, I was spending so much time on the phone one on one telling people about what I did naturally to bring about a cure and eventually realized that they weren't necessarily capable of taking it all in at once. So I decided to put it in a book where many

139

people could have access and each could read at their own pace, take time to absorb, and then pick it up again. "Why Me" isn't just about recovery from cancer; it is about living successfully – totally happy in all areas of your life... Living an exciting successful energized life!

,,

Yvonne Chamberlain, 2010.

To hear my exclusive interview with Yvonne and learn exactly what she did to kick cancer out of her life, download an audio of her amazing interview, 'Yvonne Takes On Black Melanoma and Wins!' Here: http://thegoodwitch.ca/yvonne-takes-on-black-melanoma/

All of these people took a proactive approach to healing and cured themselves. They put their old beliefs aside, and dug deep inside themselves to find the answers that were waiting there for them all along. They trusted their infinite healing wisdom.

These stories are only a handful of the thousands and thousands of stories from people who have healed themselves from all types of cancer. To hear their stories of natural healing, plus more stories of healing from all over the world, from all kinds of diseases, symptoms and syndromes, go to *www.IncredibleHealingJournals.com*.

See Yourself Healed!
Using your power is about being proactive and . . . it is about using the tools you already have!

What tools? Your mind and your body, of course! Use your mind to focus your intent on healing your body.

The fastest and easiest way to focus intent on healing is to use visualization. By seeing yourself healed, the way you want to be, you *make* it happen. You *are* in control of the healing process and that's exactly where you want to be.

Visualization is not difficult, it does not take special skills or strict methods. Visualization must be done regularly to be effective. The more you do it, the more experienced you will become and the easier it will be to bring that picture of perfect health, back to yourself.

A simple way to begin to visualize is when you lie in bed at night. It is easy to remember and be consistent. Put a small reminder, a picture or saying on a piece of paper, and tape it near where you sleep to remind

140

you of what you want to be like, without cancer, in perfect health, enjoying life, confident and happy, not stressed or worried. Get clear on exactly how you want to be, then keep that picture with you always, never let it out of your sight or mind.

Author Mary McGillis, who writes about and teaches the magic world of ancient celtic traditions, tells us when negative thoughts of illness occur, to simply grab them out of your mind with your hand, and throw them away.

It may sound strange at first, but it really works! After throwing away your negative thought, you may not be able to remember what the thought was about, even if you try! Simply motion with your hand as if you are *capturing* and *throwing* away the negative thought, then immediately replace it with an opposite, positive thought. In this way, you will quickly regain control of your healing process.

Use Active Visualization To Kill Cancer Cells

Sit or lie in a quiet place without distractions. Use meditative music, or silence if you prefer. Use different methods of *killing* your cancer cells. You may imagine a fire burning your tumor up and the dead cells being carried away by smoke, or imagine your natural killer cells, gobbling up cancerous cells, and your tumor gradually disintegrating, leaving only healthy, pink flesh behind.

If your cancer is throughout your bloodstream, imagine natural killer cells all over your body, recognizing, then destroying every cancer cell in your blood, or imagine a healing fire, engulfing your entire body, burning up only cancer cells, leaving only healthy *you* behind. Use whatever method *you* like, to kill your cancer. It does not matter how you imagine your cancer being killed, just that you do it, and *believe* it.

Apoptosis is the process by which your immune system triggers a cell to kill itself, and the cell carries through with the instructions, destroying itself in a series of cascading events. Watch this video of apoptosis by Drew Berry: *Apoptosis and Signal Transduction*. Use this animation to create your own visualization for finding, destroying and removing cancerous cells or tumors. Here: www.wehi.edu.au/education/wehitv/apoptosis_and_signal_transduction/ (spaces are underlines!)

What you are doing is using your powerful mind to focus your immune system on a particular problem; a very effective and well documented way of healing!

To learn more about visualization, and specific methods to eradicate cancer using this amazing technique, I suggest you check out Adam Dreamhealer's website. Adam is a young intellectual genius, who recently completed with highest honors, a Bachelor of Science degree in

Molecular Biology and Biochemistry and is completing his studies to be a medical doctor and a naturopathic doctor. Adam is a healer, speaker, visionary and best selling international author, with books in twenty-one languages and thirty-five countries! (Adam Dreamhealer, 2010).

I think Adam has a special way of teaching people. He strives to find scientific proof on the effectiveness of visualization in healing and runs experiments such as the 'Global Intention Heals Project.' This project records the EEG brainwave measurements of a healee, to show the connection to that individual, while people at an Intention Heals workshop focus on healing a specific problem for this person (Adam, 2010).

Many people have benefited from Adam's lessons on visualization and by his healing workshops (several of which I have been fortunate enough to attend). Adam has created a DVD which illustrates exactly how to use visualization techniques to heal yourself, *Dreamhealer: Visualizations for Self-Empowerment*. This DVD is singularly one of the greatest gifts our world has *ever* received.

For more information about Adam and how to heal with intention, visit Adam's website at *www.Dreamhealer.com*.

Now you are using your *power*. You hold a vision of yourself healed, and you use visualization regularly to kill any cancer cells in your body.

Now you know your body is a healing machine. *Are you with me?* Let's add the next principle!

37 Principle 2 ~ Cleanse and Detoxify!

Cleansing is the quickest way to rid your body of waste, toxins and pathogens like parasites and fungi, which in turn, allows it to work stronger and faster to heal itself. Your body is already continually cleansing and detoxifying but using specific cleanses can speed up the process and make you feel better faster. There are many ways to cleanse. Depending on your condition, sometimes more gentle cleanses are in order. Other times, the situation becomes so acute that an immediate cleanse is the only thing that will stop you from having a medical intervention like surgery.

To give you an example, for years I ate a rich diet with meat, fatty cheeses and butter. I gave no thought to the sticky, hydrogenated fat I was eating in my peanut butter sandwiches. I took birth control pills for ten years before I had children, not realizing that synthetic hormones were having a detrimental effect and contributing to my problems, by causing cholesterol to accumulate in my liver and gall bladder.

By the time I was in my mid-40s, excess cholesterol, hydrogenated, damaged and saturated fats and synthetic hormones had completely congested my liver and gall bladder. I had taken in way more than my liver was able to deal with, and now I was facing clogged arteries, *fatty liver* and gallstones.

I started having chronic digestive problems and constant discomfort under my right rib cage, which sometimes sent me to bed writhing in pain. My doctor ordered an ultrasound that showed no stones, so I went away, not knowing what to do. Six months later I was back in her office, after a severe gall bladder attack. I didn't know at the time, but every gall bladder attack was caused by a gallstone moving through the tiny bile duct as my body was trying desperately to remove the buildup.

The doctor pulled open my file and looked at the results of my ultrasound six months earlier, and told me I did not have gallstones, but I did have a mild case of *fatty liver*. A *mild* case to the doctor who was not experiencing the symptoms; but to me, it was disrupting my life, I was in constant discomfort and was ready to do almost anything, short of removing my gall bladder!

The problem was, I knew I was having gall bladder attacks, and I was scared because the next and only step in conventional treatment was removal of my gall bladder. I asked my doctor what help they could offer me, but her only solution was choleocystectomy, or gall bladder removal.

Many of my clients and friends, male and female, all around the same age, were having their gall bladders removed. It seemed like an epidemic. There was absolutely no way I would let surgeons remove my gall bladder. There had to be a better way.

I knew there must be a correlation to all the junk I had eaten in the past and my present condition, so I researched until I found the answer, a liver and gall bladder purge. After I did the first cleanse I felt so much better I wanted to do another one almost immediately. When you see hundreds of tiny 'gallstones' floating in the toilet, you will know immediately the cleanse has worked, and I speak from experience when I say you will be glad those gallstones are in the toilet instead of in you!

Five cleanses later, and after the expulsion of around 450 *fatty liver* stones, my digestion is now back to normal. The stones were sized anywhere from a large grain of sand to three stones that were about three quarters of an inch long! They were pea green, the same color as bile, were soft, and could be cut by a knife, almost like soft chocolate. I left several *stones* in a tiny cardboard box, to show my children, and over a short time, the stones leaked fat and the cardboard soaked it up! All that was left were deflated skins! If you are curious to see what gallstones or fatty liver deposits look like, just do a search for *'purged gallstones'* on Google Images, where there are hundreds of examples of stones that were cleansed out by using similar methods.

After the cleanses, my discomfort and pain immediately disappeared. It took several months for my digestive system to heal from the damage done by stomach acid, but now, three years later, I have no more pain, my digestion is normal, and I experience no more *acid reflux* symptoms.

This cleanse was imperative to my healing process. I needed help fast, and the Liver Gallbladder purge was my answer. It jump started my healing process!

If you are confused by the mountains of cleanses available for purchase in stores, let me help you. The best and cheapest way to cleanse is with natural foods and herbs. Do not buy expensive cleanses until you at least try your own first.

I was astounded when I heard that a woman paid $600 for liver cleanses. Supplies for the liver cleanse, of pink grapefruits, olive oil and Epsom salts cost about three dollars Canadian and the cleanse is over within twenty-four hours!

Some cleanses use herbs, which are readily available in bulk, in just about any small city, not to mention the ones that grow in your own backyard and fields around your home.

For example, Burdock grows everywhere on the farmlands of southern Ontario and is so invasive it is considered a pest, yet every part of the plant is medicinal. Specifically, Burdock is an effective blood cleanser. You will see Burdock in many commercial formulas.

Some cleanses do not use herbs, and instead use fresh raw fruits, vegetables and water, which are even easier to obtain.

The **Brown Rice Cleanse** is very effective and extremely simple; a perfect first cleanse. You will never feel deprived because there are so many foods allowed, and this cleanse makes you *feeeeel* great.

My brother was not feeling well for several months so I urged him to try the Brown Rice Cleanse. Scott stayed on this cleanse for two entire months, simply because he felt so much better!

This cleanse slowly and gently removes toxins and buildup from your organs, tissues and fluids, while simultaneously rebuilding your trillions of cells with a rich supply of easily absorbable nutrients.

LEMON JUICE/ CAYENNE CLEANSE

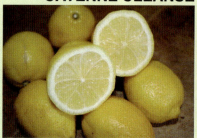

Well known as the Master Cleanser or the Lemonade Diet, this simple cleanse was made famous by Stanley Burroughs in the 1976 book, *The Master Cleanser*. It dissolves and eliminates toxins and congestion throughout your body, cleansing kidneys, liver, glands, cells, joints and muscles.

To make your own lemonade cleanse, mix the juice of half a lemon, two spoonfuls of 100% maple syrup and a pinch of cayenne pepper with a large cup of hot water.

Stanley Burroughs suggests drinking six to twelve glasses of lemonade each day, avoiding all other food and drinks, except water. He also suggests a gentle laxative herbal tea to assist in elimination of wastes released into your digestive system.

He recommends diabetics do the cleanse with molasses instead of maple syrup (Burroughs, 1976).

Brown Rice Cleanse ~ Comforting and Supportive

This is a cleanse I really enjoy doing. It is easy to follow and you never feel deprived because you can eat a huge variety of foods. It is safe and even beneficial for diabetics as it evens out sugar levels in the blood immediately!

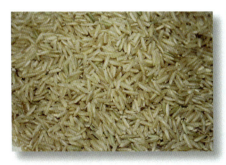

For months and months I was having constant headaches and reactions to certain foods. This happened immediately when I ate MSG, caffeine, spicy foods, sodium benzoate and a few other chemicals and preservatives. It also happened when someone sprayed perfume near me, or when I was in a stressful situation, or got emotionally worked up about something.

Clearly, I needed to detox! During these episodes, which had increased in frequency to two or three times per day, my face would go beat red, to the point where I could defrost a small ice pack in a matter of minutes from the heat on my cheeks alone! When you look at my cheeks now (even though this never happens to me now) you can see the vascular damage, where the tiny vessels underneath my skin had broken from the heat.

When I visited my doctor, she told me it was Rosacea. I asked how to stop it from happening, but she did not have an answer, and simply said it was very common. This did not make me feel any better. The headaches were tiresome, I was popping acetaminophen like crazy and my hot, red face, was embarrassing!

This cleanse was a miracle for me. It cleared up my headaches quickly, but it also proved to me that cleanses work. It told me what was really wrong and helped me to realize that even though Rosacea was common, there was an underlying problem – my body was stressed and full of junk!

After months and months of headaches, seven days on this cleanse and I could eat anything without getting a reaction. I was ecstatic, as I had not been without a headache for what seemed like ages. My poor eating habits (I thought I was eating healthy food!) caught up with me about two and a half months later. The headaches returned slowly and steadily. This was several years ago, and I have since performed many different cleanses, and eat delicious, healthy foods every day. I have not experienced symptoms for a few years now.

I think it is important to point out that this cleanse was instrumental in helping me to detoxify and heal my body, when I was just beginning my healing journey.

This cleanse is so nutritious and well-rounded that you could eat like this every day for a very long time, your whole life in fact! You can eat as much as you want, whenever you want. There is no need to count calories or weigh portions. Drink lots of fresh water and herbal tea throughout your cleanse. Be sure to fill your refrigerator with fresh, organic fruits and vegetables, grains, and snacking foods as listed below. Stay on this cleansing diet for as long as you feel like!

You may experience detoxification symptoms, including headaches, muscle and joint pain, mild digestive upset, decreased energy and changes in bowel habits. These symptoms should last for one to three days. The key to this diet is that it eliminates all allergenic and troublesome foods.

DO NOT EAT ~ Allergenic Foods

- Alcohol, Coffee, Black Tea, Soft Drinks

- Barley, Rye, Wheat, Oats (the gluten grains)

- Corn

- Beef, Pork, Shellfish

- Dairy products of all kinds

- Eggs

- Soy products

- Refined and/or processed foods, (white flour, white rice or sugar)

- Yeast containing foods

- Chocolate

- Oranges

EAT AS MUCH AS YOU LIKE AND ORGANIC WHEREVER POSSIBLE!

Proteins
- Organic or farm fresh, chicken, turkey or lamb
- Wild cold water fish such as salmon, tuna and cod
- Chick peas, lima beans, kidney beans, navy beans, adzuki beans, pinto beans
- Red, green, black or orange lentils

Beverages
- Mineral or spring water
- Fresh unsweetened juices – vegetable or fruit, diluted half with water
- Herbal teas
- Rice milk
- Almond, cashew, coconut, hazelnut or macadamia nut milk
- Hemp, sunflower seed or pumpkin seed milk

Fruits

- Apples, apricots, bananas, blueberries, cherries, grapes, kiwi, lemons, mango, papaya, peaches, pears, pineapple, plums, raspberries, strawberries, pomegranates
- Dried fruits, organic, non-sulphured

Vegetables
- Alfalfa sprouts, artichoke, asparagus, avocado, yellow and green beans
- Beets, beet greens, carrots, red, green or yellow sweet peppers, celery, cucumber
- Bok choy, broccoli, brussel sprouts, cabbage, cauliflower, kale, eggplant, endive, escarole, kohlrabi, leeks
- Romaine, Boston, leaf or iceberg lettuce, spinach, Swiss chard

- Okra, onions, parsley, parsnips, peas, potatoes, radishes, rutabaga, snow peas

- Winter squash (acorn, butternut, spaghetti), Summer squash (zucchini), sweet potatoes, taro

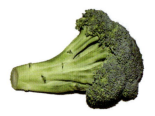

- Tomatoes, turnips, water chestnuts, watercress, mushrooms

Grains
- Brown rice, brown rice cakes, whole grain rice crackers, whole grain rice cereal, whole grain rice noodles, brown rice bread

- Amaranth, Millet, Quinoa

Raw Nuts and Seeds
- Almonds, cashews, pecans, pine, macadamia, walnuts

- Poppy, hemp, pumpkin, sesame, sunflower seeds, flax

Oils
Keep oils refrigerated. Do not use for cooking. For cooking use coconut oil or ghee (clarified butter). Use olive oil or sesame oil with broth, stock or water.
- Cold pressed organic flax seed oil

- Olive oil, sesame oil, sunflower oil, hemp oil

Herbs and Spices
- Fresh garlic, ginger and onion

- Fresh or dried cayenne, paprika, turmeric and chili

- Fresh or dried herbs, such as dill, coriander, parsley, mint, sage, rosemary, thyme, oregano, tarragon

- Sea salt – unrefined only or Herbamare

- Non-salt herbal seasoning or Mrs. Dash

Sweeteners
- Raw or unpasteurized organic honey, maple syrup, brown rice syrup or raw agave nectar

- Blended dried fruits, date sugar, stevia

You will feel light and refreshed after several days with only nutritional, supportive and cleansing foods. After your cleanse reintroduce allergenic foods one at a time, paying close attention to any reactions you may have to a particular food. If your pulse rate increases when you reintroduce pork, for example, it could mean a food sensitivity. This can cause stress on your system and an inability to digest and assimilate this food.

You may return to the Brown Rice Cleanse anytime you feel congested or "toxinated." Pay close attention to your symptoms and your body will tell you when it is ready for your next cleanse.

For more cleansing information, and more cleanses, go to *Cleanse Your Body*, where you will find the Water Cleanse, Lemon Juice Cleanse, Watermelon Cleanse, Raw Vegan Cleanse and more, nine cleanses in all, starting simple and working up to the more complex Gall Bladder Liver Purge. Here: www.thegoodwitch.ca/start-with-cleanses-first/

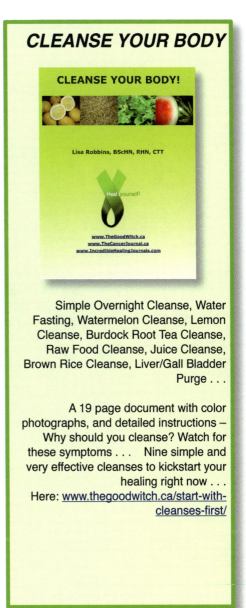

CLEANSE YOUR BODY

CLEANSE YOUR BODY!

Lisa Robbins, BScHN, RHN, CTT

Heal yourself!

www.TheGoodWitch.ca
www.TheCancerJournal.ca
www.IncredibleHealingJournals.com

Simple Overnight Cleanse, Water Fasting, Watermelon Cleanse, Lemon Cleanse, Burdock Root Tea Cleanse, Raw Food Cleanse, Juice Cleanse, Brown Rice Cleanse, Liver/Gall Bladder Purge . . .

A 19 page document with color photographs, and detailed instructions – Why should you cleanse? Watch for these symptoms . . . Nine simple and very effective cleanses to kickstart your healing right now . . .
Here: www.thegoodwitch.ca/start-with-cleanses-first/

Now that you are using your *power* and truly know you are a healing machine, and you have started to *cleanse* and *detoxify* your body, you are ready for the next principle.

38   Principle 3 ~ Super Nutrition!

What is super nutrition?

It is food that is not just *good* for you, it is food that quickly and easily thrusts your body into healing mode. It is food that tastes amazing and fresh, and makes you *feeeeel* super! Natural, whole foods provide the building blocks for your beautiful human body. The more natural, the closer to their whole state, the better.

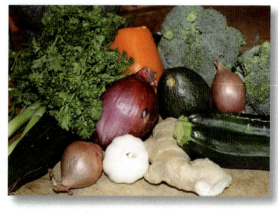

An apple plucked fresh from a tree, organic asparagus poking tiny heads up to the sun in early spring, dandelion leaves picked first thing, in the moist, early morning, or tiny red clover sprouts, bursting with nutrients at only four days old; these are whole, natural foods with super nutrition. Nothing suits our bodies better!

Super nutrition is food that is unprocessed, without chemicals or additives of any kind. Food that is grown naturally, organically. Think dark brown organic apricots, dried slowly in the sun, instead of bright orange, artificially dehydrated, pesticide laden apricots, preserved with sulphur dioxide. It seems almost surreal to be concerned about carcinogens in the most basic of all needs, our food. The best way to avoid hormones, pesticides and foods with added chemicals is to buy raw, organic food from reputable suppliers.

You can grow your own vegetables and fruits at home in your garden too. It is also very simple to grow culinary herbs like thyme, sage and oregano or medicinal herbs such as burdock, red clover or motherwort in your home garden. How? Just plant them!

Organic produce is everywhere now, at farmers' markets and grocery stores and most times the prices are only slightly higher than their non-organic counterparts. If you replace packaged and processed foods with organic produce, your grocery bill most likely, will not be any higher than before.

Buying a bag of organic sweet potatoes and cutting them into sticks is much cheaper and will feed more people, than purchasing a frozen bag of already sliced non-organic sweet potatoes! Mashed potatoes in a box? The same price as a ten pound bag of fresh potatoes from a local farmer who grows organically. See what I mean?

Buying from local suppliers and farmers supports your local organic farming community, keeps our environment healthy, and sends a powerful message to food suppliers:

We want safe and healthy food and we will pay more and go to more trouble to get it!

We, the collective population, 2010.

Rehydrate With Water

Nutrition would not be super without water! We all know we need water to survive, but how much is enough? The answer is simple. Drink water whenever you are thirsty and drink until you feel well hydrated. Pay particular attention to your lips, mouth and skin as they show signs of dehydration quickly. It is easy to become dehydrated in dry weather, especially if you are not paying attention to your body's messages.

Adequate water intake helps your kidneys flush out toxins and wastes. Symptoms of dehydration include headaches, constipation, joint problems, fatigue, difficulty concentrating, flashes from overheating, dry skin, mouth or lips, frequent infections and dry, brittle hair (Holford, 2004).

Excessive amounts of water can cause leaching of magnesium and other nutrients. Patrick Holford, founder of the Institute For Optimum Nutrition and author of *The New Optimum Nutrition Bible* writes, "more than 1.5 to 2 quarts per day can tax the kidneys and lead to over-hydration. Taken to the extreme, this can kill you" (Holford, 2004).

Always carry water with you, preferably in a stainless steel or glass container. If you drink water from a city supply, filter it, then fill a jug and place in the refrigerator or on the counter, to release chlorine gas before drinking.

Drink fresh spring or mineral water whenever possible. The minerals in these waters help to re-alkalize your body. Distilled water can leach minerals from your body; better choices are spring, mineral, well or filtered tap water.

Whole Foods

Eat foods that are as close as possible to their natural raw state. For example on a scale of processing, consider the oat:

Raw – Dried oat groats – soaked
Natural Cooked oat groats – Irish Oatmeal cereal
Slightly Processed – Steel cut oats – whole oat squashed flat
Processed – Regular oats – sliced and squashed flat
Highly Processed – Quick cook oats – sliced thinly – cooked and squashed flat
Refined – Instant oats – very thin – cooked – high in carbohydrates – low in nutrients – cook instantly

Cut Out The Sugar

Cutting back on sugar and refined carbohydrates makes it difficult for cancer to grow. Sugar is the perfect yeast food. Think bread-making, yeast, warm water and sugar; fermenting, foaming and bubbling as the yeast eat, grow, release gases and reproduce.

Sugar feeds cancer – it's as simple as that!

HEADACHES AND WATER

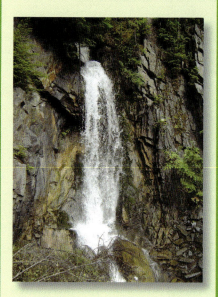

Headaches are often caused by dehydration. If you have a headache, before reaching for a pain pill, try a large glass of water first and wait ten minutes. If you still have a headache you can try a Magnesium supplement (headaches can be a symptom of a Magnesium deficiency) which helps to relax muscles and relieve tension.

Try chewing on a few Feverfew leaves, from the plant in your garden. You do have Feverfew in your garden don't you? It is a very useful plant!

If your headache is caused by tension or stress, try a calming blend of lavender and chamomile tea. Buy the tea loose and blend or use a teabag of each kind, to make a full pot of tea. Combined, these therapies can clear the worst of headaches without stressing your liver with the job of detoxifying every molecule of medication!

If you want to starve cancer:

- **Never** eat high fructose corn syrup, like found in sodas and commercially prepared iced teas and other beverages. Instead, make your own iced tea with herbal fruit tea bags, like blueberry, cherry or raspberry, fresh lemon juice, stevia or raw agave syrup and water . . . You will never buy commercial iced tea again!
- **Drastically** limit your consumption of sugar, sweets, cakes, pies, cookies, sweet sauces and alcohol. Replace them with fresh raw fruits, dried fruits, and delicious raw desserts, like the ones in *Ani's Raw Food Desserts - 85 Easy, Delectable Sweet Treats*! Here: www.thegoodwitch.ca/bookshelf/
- **Eliminate** processed white bread, white rice and other high glycemic carbohydrate foods and replace them with whole grains like brown basmati rice, quinoa and millet, and whole grain breads in moderation. Eat two to three fresh, raw fruits every day, focussing on the anti-angiogenic fruits (possessing properties that cut off blood supply which feeds tumors), such as apples, berries, oranges, lemons, grapefruits, red grapes, pomegranates, peaches, cherries and cranberries.

Focus on Sea Vegetables

When I was a kid growing up, I used to think that milk was *nature's most perfect food*. I am not sure where I got this idea, but it might have had something to do with the milk mustache . . .

Now, I am all grown up, and I *know* the most perfect food, the ultimate superfood, is *seaweed*!

Sea vegetables are our richest source of nutrients. *Seaweed* has everything! Really . . . in nutritional profiles, seaweed outweighs every other food for content of vitamins, minerals, trace elements and phytochemicals. Seaweeds are high in anti-angiogenic properties, helping to reduce cancerous growths by cutting off their blood supply. Coastal people *know* that seaweeds are a rich source of minerals, and eat them every day to stay beautiful, healthy and have a long life.

Seaweeds are a rich source of iodine, a nutrient essential for the manufacture of thyroid hormones. A deficiency in iodine is the most common cause of goiter or enlargement of the thyroid gland in humans, but sadly, this deficiency is often overlooked. Most North American soils are depleted of iodine, which was added to table salt to reduce deficiencies and high incidences of goiter, early in the 20th century. Seaweeds are known to detoxify your body, preventing the accumulation of heavy metals and environmental toxins.

Seaweeds have been studied extensively for their anti-cancer and anti-tumor properties. Their nutrients are available and useable when the seaweeds are eaten raw, but many are damaged by cooking, including fluorine and most vitamins. Fluorine is an important nutrient for bone

154

and teeth health, and is not the same as fluoride, which is a byproduct of the aluminum smelting industry (Bowden, 2007).

There are currently many studies of seaweeds because the pharmaceutical industries want to extract what they think is the active anti-cancer component . . . to make a new drug . . . that is patented. We *know* that eating seaweed gives you all the anti-cancer components and nutrients that your body needs to repair itself and we are quite capable of extracting the anti-cancer compounds ourselves! *Are you with me?*

Add raw seaweeds to your diet every day. How? You can start by making your own sushi with raw nori sheets. I know of only two suppliers of raw nori in my area, but roasted nori is everywhere. You can also just eat a piece of raw nori by itself as a snack or use it to make veggie rolls. Put half an avocado, sprouts, tomato slices, greens like lettuce or spinach, and a dribble of your favorite salad dressing in the middle of a sheet of nori. Fold up the bottom, then roll the sides into a cone shape and eat immediately, before the nori has a chance to become soft.

Buy raw seaweed flakes, and add to salads and vegetable juices or sprinkle them into soups and stews. Adding them *after* cooking retains the quality of their nutrients.

Miso soup is simple to make with fermented white miso, from the refrigerator section of your health food store. Just add 1 to 2 tablespoons of white miso to your favorite big cup, pour in boiling water and throw in a few pieces of raw wakame or kombu seaweed. Add several cubes of *organic* firm tofu (always eat your tofu organic!). Allow the seaweed to soften and soak up the broth. Relax and enjoy this salty, nutritious treat.

For more information about Miso Soup and Macrobiotic eating, see *Miso Soup Recipe* at www.TheGoodWitch.ca. Here: www.thegoodwitch.ca/miso-soup-recipe/

There is no family of foods more protective against radiation and environmental pollutants than sea vegetables.

Steven Schecter, Naturopathic Doctor.

Grow Your Own Sprouts

Sprouts are a mini nutrition powerhouse. All the nutrients needed to feed a growing plant are available in a tiny sprout. They are a rich source of protein, live enzymes, vitamins, minerals, phytochemicals and cancer fighting chemicals.

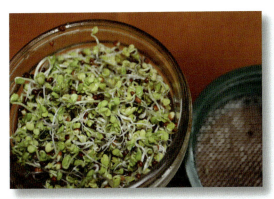

Broccoli and other cruciferous sprouts contain significant amounts of important cancer fighting compounds including sulforaphane and indole 3 carbinol, known for protecting against all cancers, but providing special protection against cancers in hormonal tissues, like breast, cervix and prostate. These natural chemicals are known to induce apoptosis (self-destruction) in cancer cells and increase the production of protective, free radical fighting enzymes (Bowden, 2007).

A study on extracts of three-day-old broccoli sprouts concluded they were highly effective in reducing the incidence, multiplication and development of chemically induced mammary tumors in rats. The authors stated, "Small quantities of crucifer sprouts may protect against the risk of cancer as effectively as much larger quantities of mature vegetables of the same variety."

The study showed that three-day-old broccoli and cauliflower sprouts contained anywhere from ten to one hundred times the levels of sulforaphane than whole plants of the same kind! (Fahey, Zhang, Talalay, 1997).

Making your own sprouts is super easy with a sprouting lid and glass jar. The lid has tiny holes to rinse the seeds, and let air in. Your health food store will carry lids, jars and seeds for sprouting, like broccoli, red clover, fennel and onion seeds. It is handy to have two, (or up to four for a family) sprouting jars and lids, so one can be sprouting, while the other is being eaten! Red Clover seeds are ready to eat in five days from soaking, and are perfect for your first sprouting adventure. Soak the seeds overnight in the jar, then rinse and leave upside down to drain. Rinse the seeds twice per day until they are fully sprouted, then move the jar to the refrigerator.

You can grow delicious, crunchy, sweet pea shoots in a tray or pot. Plant them really close together in loose potting soil, place them in the sun, water and wait. When the shoots are three inches tall, cut them off with scissors and throw them into your salad or smoothie. The plants will not revive after cutting so you must plant more seeds for more shoots.

Never eat sprouts from seeds that have been treated with fungicides, which you can see and smell on the seeds! Get used to smelling your food. You can detect fungicides and herbicides on most produce at small levels. Next time you are at the grocery store, smell a bag of organic potatoes, then smell a bag of regular potatoes. You will notice the difference immediately.

Make Juice

Fresh juice infuses you with life. It raises your vibration. Live vegetable and fruit juices supply a host of vitamins, minerals, phytochemicals, and live enzymes that protect your body against damage by carcinogens and pathogens. Fresh juices provide the basic materials your body systems need to function perfectly. Most importantly, they provide your immune system with the tools it needs to fight illness.

Many people report using juicing to successfully slow down, stop and even reverse the growth of cancers. Remember Jay Kordich, The Juice Daddy? He was diagnosed with bladder cancer at the age of twenty-five. He enlisted the help of the famous cancer healer, Max Gerson, who immediately put him on a juice diet. Now he is eighty-six and healthy as an ox! By juicing fresh vegetables and fruit, Jay cured himself!

Drink at least two glasses of fresh vegetable juice daily. Use a good quality juice extractor. Concentrate on vegetables such as carrots, celery, broccoli, cabbage, cauliflower, cucumber, asparagus, kale, spinach and beets. Add apples for sweetness and added nutrients. Add a thumb size hunk of ginger, or dried spices such as cinnamon, nutmeg or cardamom to your fresh juices for flavor and a boost in antioxidant protection.

Try Cleansing Green Juice for a detoxifying, alkalizing and supportive juice, with liver and blood cleansing benefits, also helpful for weight loss. The white pith from lemons helps to break up kidney and gallbladder stones. The ingredients are common and the juice is simple and quick to make: Juice one celery stalk, one large carrot, one cucumber and two apples.

Add this juice to a blender with one large handful of leafy greens. Vary your greens as you like or as is available: asparagus, spinach, kale, chard, beet greens, collard, arugula, lettuce, watercress, parsley, or coriander. Add one large thumb-size hunk of fresh ginger root and quarter of a fresh lemon, skin removed, with some pith left in place. Blend and serve.

This juice is very suitable for diabetics when taken between regular meals and can be watered down as much as needed.

Drink Smoothies

Smoothies are a fast and delicious way to add raw foods to your diet. They are so easy to make and taste so great you will want one at least once a day, even better, twice a day.

Have fun adding fresh or frozen fruits, ground flax seeds or flax oil and vegetables like celery. If you have no fresh raw greens on hand, keep dried kale flakes or a bottle of green supplement to add to your smoothies when needed. Rich dark greens provide an abundance of the nutrients lacking in most people's diets, including those involved in immunity and defense. Focus on green.

I started making green smoothies for breakfast to help me go more *raw*. The first time I offered a green smoothie to my husband Bob, he turned up his nose, but tried it anyway. Now I have to make enough for him, my three kids and all their friends.

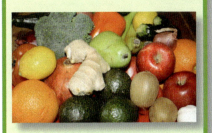

PSORIASIS AND ECZEMA

These conditions are a clue from your body that your blood is too sweet and acidic. They can be healed by cleansing your body, and choosing fresh, delicious and nutritious foods, and by completely eliminating sugar and refined carbohydrates from your diet.

If I go a morning without a smoothie and make something else, my husband Bob starts complaining that he is hungry. I laughed my head off when I heard him explaining to his friends, how good he feels after drinking a green smoothie! Believe me . . . he is about as old as a dinosaur and about as stubborn, and even he knows how good a green smoothie makes him *feeeeel*!

Make sure it is green with Swiss chard, kale, asparagus, spinach or dark lettuce, and creamy with a handful of raw nuts or seeds. That way the smoothie replenishes you – an instant liquid meal of nourishing essential fats, carbohydrates, protein, vitamins, minerals and phytochemicals. A banana, a handful of greens, a handful of raw nuts or seeds (or flax or hemp oil), water and if you want, a thumb size nob of ginger for a little extra bam.

Need more? Meet Victoria Boutenko and the Raw Family. She is considered the *guru* of green smoothies and going raw. Their new book *Fresh* is my personal favorite with the most delicious raw food recipes, including Almond Cake; a perfect dessert if only by merit of flavour alone, a fresh burst of orange in rich date, carob and ground almonds, crisped up with dripping sweet and sour lemon glaze . . . full raw . . . one-hundred percent, cancer fighting nutrition. Here: www.thegoodwitch.ca/bookshelf/

Here are some more ideas . . .

Try the 'Basic Green Smoothie'. My favorite variation on the basic green smoothie is the 'Chai Green Smoothie.' Or try the 'Orange Banana Smoothie,' at TheGoodWitch.ca. Here: www.thegoodwitch.ca/category/nutrition/ or use the search bar and type in smoothie.

Eat More Raw Foods

Eating raw foods provides optimum nutrients. Why cook the nutrients out of your food, then pay money for nutritional supplements? Eat your food raw every possible chance you get.

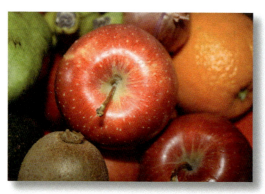

Instead of cooking asparagus into a limp, nutrient deficient flop, add fresh, delicious, raw asparagus to your salad.

Instead of baking cookies, try mashing bananas and sprinkling in cinnamon. Spoon onto parchment paper and dehydrate into raw banana cinnamon cookies.

Instead of pasteurized juice, eat a piece of seasonal fruit; sweet, juicy and fresh; a whole orange instead of *cooked* (pasteurized) orange juice. Add the juice of one fresh orange to a tall glass of water with ice for a refreshing drink. Chop small pieces of fresh lemon and keep in the refrigerator to add to water anytime.

Instead of pasteurized cranberry juice from a carton or jar, try making your own raw refreshing, 'Cranberry Cleanser' with your blender. You only need to keep frozen cranberries on hand to always have your own supply of fresh and delicious Cranberry juice. Here: www.thegoodwitch.ca/cranberry-cleanser/

Steam your vegetables so lightly, they are mostly raw. Order maki rolls with raw vegetables like cucumber, avocado and asparagus.

Add your vegetables in the last couple of minutes of cooking time, or chop them really tiny and add completely raw after cooking. Scrambled eggs are delicious with raw, finely chopped shallots, tomatoes, broccoli and coriander, added just before serving. Always add fresh raw herbs *after* cooking.

Grow your own delicious fresh sprouts in a few days!

Eat more salads! For some delicious additions to salad, and some classic, rocking salad dressings, check out *Salad Strategies*, which covers Salad Toppings, Basic Vinaigrette, Basic Balsamic, Sweet Honey Dijon Vinaigrette, Vivacious Vinaigrette, Fabulous French, Gorgeous Greek Salad and Gorgeous Greek Pasta Salad. Here: www.thegoodwitch.ca/salad-strategies/

Buy a raw food book from favorite raw food chefs, The Raw Family or Ani Phyo. Many of my raw recipes are derived from their amazing, original creations. See www.thegoodwitch.ca/bookshelf/

Try *Raw Nut and Dried Fruit Nosh*, or trail mix made with your favorite raw, organic, nuts, seeds and naturally dried fruit. Here: www.thegoodwitch.ca/raw-nut-and-dried-fruit-nosh/

Make lots, keep it refrigerated, and eat some every day! Mix it up and try new ingredients each time.

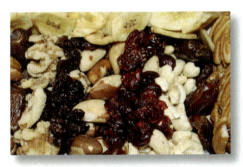

The point is to make raw food more a part of your life. Gradually make the shift and tip the balance. No one has to be 100% raw, and many do not believe it is necessary, but the closer to a whole raw diet, the better. In a world where we are brought up on comforting warm, cooked food, it is difficult to give up everything we are used to, like hot, garlic, mashed potatoes with butter, or piping hot broccoli cheddar soup on a cold autumn day. Know that you never have to give up anything. You can eat whatever you want, in moderation; well, except for hydrogenated fat – you still can't eat that!

I was given a book recently by my friend's mother. Mrs. McLean told David, "this will just get thrown out after I'm gone, so you might as well give it to Lisa because I know she will read it." Mrs. McLean's father Morgan was one of seven children. All the children died early in life, except for one, Morgan. In 1978, Morgan bought a book called, *The Miracle of Live Juices and Raw Foods*, written by John H. Tobe in 1977. He followed the regimen outlined in the book for the remainder of his life, and out of seven children, Morgan was the only one who lived well into his nineties!

Cooked foods are hard to digest, requiring extra digestive enzymes which must be produced by your pancreas. Raw foods come prepackaged with live digestive enzymes, which help to break down the food particles, releasing their nutrients without added stress on you or your digestive system.

The doctor of the future will no longer treat the human frame with drugs, but rather will cure and prevent disease with nutrition.

Thomas Edison

Can you imagine an apple sitting on your counter for a long time, say three months? The apple would become riper and riper, then gradually shrivel up and digest itself. Now, imagine cooking that apple, then leaving the cooked apple on the counter for the same amount of time. The apple can no longer ripen, or digest itself. It does not break down or ferment. Instead, mold settles on the outside of the apple, and begins to grow, taking over the apple.

Many people have used raw foods to cure disease.

Healing Cancer From The Inside Out, is a book and documentary film, featuring testimonials of people who have cured themselves using *The Rave Diet*, a raw food diet. See the Resources section at the back of this book for links.

Watch a trailer for the movie, where Mariana Pina-Bergtold and Brenda Cobb, talk about how they were pressured by doctors to have chemotherapy, radiation and surgery, but instead chose to heal themselves quickly and safely using raw foods. Here: http://www.youtube.com/watch?v=_xkyMAYmrQY

The Rave Diet is outlined in *The Rave Diet & Lifestyle book*. See the Resources section at the back of this book.

Highly Unsaturated Fats
Organic, raw, nuts, seeds and avocados are a rich source of nutrients, including *immune* boosting fats. They feed every cell in your body and are an integral part of your brain, joints, glands, and sensory organs. Omega 3 fat or linolenic acid *boosts immunity*, improves your

161

metabolism, fortifies cell integrity, expands your brain power and heightens your sense of wellbeing.

Flax seeds and wild fish liver oils are rich in Omega 3 fats and cofactor nutrients that feed your immune system and stabilize your blood sugar levels. Flax seeds are a valuable source of lignans, or phytoestrogens, important plant hormones which balance your glandular and reproductive systems, keeping you calm, happy and healthy (Erasmus, 1993).

Johanna Budwig

Until her death in 2003, at the age of ninety-five, Johanna Budwig, a German born scientist and biochemist, was considered the world's leading expert on dietary fats and oils.

In 1952, she was the central government's senior expert both for fats and pharmaceutical drugs.

On November 2, 1959, Johanna delivered a lecture, which was later printed in a book, and became an international bestseller, *Flax Oil As A True Aid For Arthritis, Heart Infarction, Cancer and Other Diseases.* The front cover of her book states that she was nominated for the Nobel prize seven times for her scientific work with highly unsaturated fats and the human body. Thousands of patients, even taken from the brink of death, have been cured by Johanna Budwig's Flax Oil and Cottage Cheese protocol (Budwig, 1994).

Dr. Budwig suggests that improper fat metabolism is at the crux of all chronic illness, and when processed, solidified or heat-treated oils are removed from the diet, glandular secretion improves dramatically and quickly, as do all functions of the body.

FLAX SEED OIL & COTTAGE CHEESE PROTOCOL

Buy fresh flax seed oil, from the refrigerator section of your Health Food Store. Check the date to be sure it is current. (If it smells distasteful, it is not fresh - Your nose knows!) Mix two tablespoons of quark or cottage cheese to one tablespoon of oil. Thoroughly mix the oil and cottage cheese until it is smooth and well combined. Take two to three times per day, depending on the severity of your condition.

Tip: Quark does not keep long, but you can freeze tiny cubes of it. Try to get Quark or Cottage Cheese made from raw unpasteurized milk products. It is difficult to source but the undamaged cysteine (protein) is of the highest quality and very beneficial in manufacturing glutathione, the master antioxidant responsible for cell defense.

Saturated, hydrogenated and damaged fats no longer have their field of electrons, necessary for recharging the cells of your body, brain and

162

nerves. When we ingest heated, solidified, otherwise damaged fats and do not eat the essential, highly unsaturated fats, like flax and hemp oil, our cells do not function properly and we become congested and diseased (Budwig, 1994).

Essential highly unsaturated fats in unprocessed, raw, liquid plant and fish oils contain highly reactive electrons, as they are alive! They are also essential for oxygen metabolism, tissue repair and rebuilding (Budwig, 1994).

Mixing cottage cheese, rich in amino acids (protein building blocks) with highly unsaturated vegetable and seed oils, such as flax oil, facilitates the water solubility of fats, enabling them to combine with protein, thus raising the level of vital functioning throughout every one of your body's trillions of cells (Budwig, 1994).

The oil and protein intake which I advise consists of mainly the most active fat I know - flax seed oil - in easily digestible form accompanied by cottage cheese . . . This simple food revises the stagnated growth processes thereby naturally causing the tumour or tumours present to dissolve and the whole range of symptoms which indicate a "dead battery" are cured. In a short time the patient feels well again. It is preferable however, not to wait until three or four doctors have pronounced a tumour as incurable - but rather your principle task is to recover your health completely by optimal nutrition.

Budwig, 1994.

Udo Erasmus

Some important points about fat from the guru of fats, Udo Erasmus, and his unequalled and exhaustive resource and best-selling book, *Fats that Heal Fats that Kill.*

All fats are made of a backbone of glycerol. Our body can join two glycerol molecules to form glucose, or our body can split a glucose molecule into two glycerol molecules to make fat. Saturated fats form a part of all membranes but are mostly used by the body as fuel. In order for fats to be burnt as fuel inside the mitochondria of your muscle cells, it must be carried into the cell first by a molecule of carnitine. Carnitine is an amino acid manufactured by your body from precursor amino acids, lysine and methionine, both readily available in meat, dairy and plant proteins.

Butter and coconut burn quicker and easier because they are mostly short chain fatty acids, unlike beef and pork which are mostly comprised of long chain fatty acids, which take longer to burn (Erasmus, 1993).

When you eat too much sugar or too many carbohydrates, there will be too many glucose molecules floating in your blood. To get the sugar out of your blood and safely stored away, your body will quickly separate these glucose molecules and transform them into saturated fat, storing them away in blatantly obvious places, like your abdomen, thighs and upper arms . . .

Humans lack the ability to process saturated fats into alpha-linolenic acid and linoleic acid, the omega 3 and 6 fats, so they must be taken in directly from foods, and this is why they are referred to as *essential* fatty acids. They are *essential* to our diets because we cannot produce them ourselves.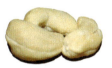

Essential Fatty Acids, or EFA's stimulate your metabolism and speed up the rate at which your body burns fat and glucose. Udo Erasmus suggests using upwards of three tablespoons per day to burn off excess fats, and help your body retain an optimal weight. Monounsaturated fats, like those found in olive oil, are used in cell membranes, and as fuel for your body (Erasmus, 1993).

Vitamins and minerals are cofactors for fat metabolism. Your body needs them to burn fat for energy. If you are deficient in any of these additional nutrients, certain functions cannot be performed and many organs and systems in your body will suffer, leading to illness and disease.

Cancer, the enigma of our time, eludes every attempt to pinpoint a single cause. It often involves fatty degeneration, something gone haywire with the way cells handle fats and energy production . . . There may be changes in the fat

*composition of cell membranes, there may be fat droplets
within cells, there may be fats surrounding tumors.*

"

Udo Erasmus, 1993.

Trans fats are produced in the processing of fats and oils, which causes a
twist in the molecule into an unnatural shape, or trans-configuration.
Udo Erasmus says, "now the molecule has its *head on backwards*, which
causes significant effects on the properties and functions of these trans
fatty molecules." The twisted shape can only partially fit into enzyme and
cell membrane structures, blocking out natural fats, while not
performing the important work needed by the fat molecules.

Trans fats are more sticky than natural fats, they cause permeability
problems in cell membranes, they burn slower in heart muscle which
normally burns EFA's, cause electrical short-circuits because of damaged
electron fields, impair your energy flow and effect all functions of your
body including your heartbeat, brain and nerve communication, your
senses and mental ability and the vitality of your body (Erasmus, 1993).

Trans fatty acids are a hideous and secret killer, sucking the life out of
you and every cell in your body. Where do they come from? Udo reports
95% of our trans fatty acid intake in Canada and the U.S. comes from
partially hydrogenated vegetable oil products (Erasmus, 1993).

Partially hydrogenated vegetable oil is used in margarine, shortening and
partially or fully hydrogenated oils. In short, it is used in most packaged
and processed foods like crackers, cookies, pastries, cakes and fast foods.

Check labels for names such as shortening, hydrogenated canola oil,
partially hydrogenated soybean oil, modified palm oil, etc.

Use healthy fats every day, but stir them in *after* your dish is cooked, to
avoid damaging the delicate fat molecules with heat. If you *have* to fry
foods, add water or vegetables to the pan first to keep the temperature
down, and protect the fats from extensive damage.

Cook with coconut fat, or a combination of olive with stock, broth or
water or organic butter or ghee, or clarified butter.

Other healthy fats include avocado, unrefined flax, sesame, hemp,
sunflower, walnut and pumpkin seed oils, and these delicate fats should
never be heated.

165

Increase your essential fatty acid intake by making yourself fresh 'Seed and Nut Milks' and store in a sealed glass jar in the refrigerator for one or two days. Add delicious, creamy nut milk to raw oatmeal, use in coffee or tea, or add to cream soups or smoothies. Here: www.thegoodwitch.ca/hemp-milk/

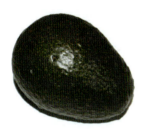

Make yourself a sumptuous mocha with fresh coffee or grain coffee, fresh raw nut milk of your choice, one teaspoon of raw cocoa powder, and a *tiny* squirt of raw agave nectar or unpasteurized honey. Then sit back, relax and visualize yourself healthy!

Another simple way to add essential fats to your diet is to make your own nutritious and delicious salad dressings. Once you realize how quick and simple it is to make your own dressings, you will never go back to store bought! Here are some basic ideas and staple recipes . . . *Salad Strategies*. Here: www.thegoodwitch.ca/salad-strategies/

Macrobiotic Diet

Linda Devine used the Macrobiotic diet to cure herself of breast cancer in only ten months. Many others have used the Macrobiotic Diet to cure a variety of illnesses, including cancer.

The term Macrobiotics was created by Hippocrates, the ancient Greek physician we know as The Father of Western Medicine. He used the term to describe people who lived long, healthy lives. The Greek translation of *macrobiotics* means *great* or *large life*.

People, all over the world, have practiced this simple way of eating and living for thousands of years. It is considered one of the most effective ways to bring balance and harmony back to your body and life. The Macrobiotic theory suggests that illness and unhappiness result when we are removed from nature and do not live in harmony with the world around us.

The Macrobiotic diet uses traditional foods like organic whole grains, mineral rich sea vegetables, locally grown seasonal vegetables and fruits, unrefined sea salt, natural sweeteners and moderate amounts of high quality protein from white fish, shellfish, and naturally prepared soy foods.

Macrobiotic chefs take much pride in preparing food for others, realizing the great responsibility they have for preparing foods in a way that directs the health and happiness of the people who will eat their nutritious creations (Esko, 1978).

In *The Macrobiotic Way, The Definitive Guide to Macrobiotic Living*, Michio Kushi, founder of the world's renowned macrobiotic educational center, the Kushi Institute, describes the standard macrobiotic diet, "50 to 60 percent whole grains, 20 to 30 percent local, organic vegetables, 5 to 10 percent beans and sea vegetables, including soy foods, 5 to 10 percent wholesome soups, and 5 percent supplementary foods including fish, desserts and beverages" (Kushi, 2004).

The Chinese philosophy of Yin and Yang, or universal balance, is at the heart of the Macrobiotic diet. Yin represents *expansion* and includes sugar, fruits, leafy green vegetables, nuts, seeds, root vegetables, beans, pork and milk. In contrast, wheat, buckwheat, rice, corn, fish, cheese, beef, eggs, and poultry are Yang foods, representing *contraction* (Kushi, 2004).

The Macrobiotic diet is made up of whole, natural foods that are neither too expansive (yin) nor too contractive (yang). Sugar for instance is at the extreme end of Yin. Cheese, beef, poultry and eggs are at the extreme end of Yang. Eating foods on the extreme end of Yin or Yang causes imbalance, and cravings for the opposite extreme. This explains why eating yang meats, eggs and salty cheeses promotes cravings for sweet foods, alcohol and coffee – all yin foods (Kushi, 2004).

How does the macrobiotic diet heal your body from cancer and other illnesses? It cleanses, rejuvenates and rebuilds worn out tissues and organs. It heals your body with nourishing and satisfying whole foods. It makes you *feeeeel* well.

If you are interested in adding more macrobiotic foods to your life, the best resource and cookbook is Michio Kushi's, *The Macrobiotic Way, The Definitive Guide To Macrobiotic Living*. This book if full of recipes, tips, tools and techniques and Michio Kushi is the ultimate Macrobiotic teacher and guru!

Protective Foods

Do you remember Dr. Duke? On the next page, you'll find the results of a search in Dr. Duke's *Phytochemical and Ethnobotanical Database* of, 'Number of Chemicals in Plants with **Anti-Tumor** Activity' (Dr. Duke's *Phytochemical and Ethnobotanical Database*, 1998).

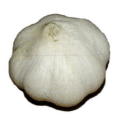

As you will see, these are regular plant foods, many we eat every day, like carrots, cauliflower, garlic, onions, tomatoes and fresh herbs. You can click on any food and go directly to Dr. Duke's database. Take note of how many different chemicals, scientists have identified specifically with *anti-tumor* activity (Dr. Duke's *Phytochemical and Ethnobotanical Database*, 1998).

Eating a variety of organic foods, prepared in a way that preserves their medicinal and nutritive properties, will protect your body with an impenetrable army of anti-cancer phytochemicals.

What is the best way to prepare our foods to retain their nutritional and medicinal properties? By leaving them raw, of course!

Raw garlic and onions are rich in many nutrients that fight cancer and boost immunity. They work better if taken fresh, not cooked.

Supplement forms can be almost as effective as fresh, especially Allicin rich garlic pills. Chop a garlic clove into tiny pieces and drink down with water. Use raw garlic and onions regularly in salads, rice and potato dishes and casseroles.

Pay attention to your body, know what it likes, what makes it *feeeeel* great, what *feeeds* it, and add *more* of those foods, and *less* of the foods that make it *feeeeel* bad!

FOOD PLANTS WITH Anti-Tumor ACTIVITY

Carrot Root - 27 chemicals
Fennel Fruit - 22 chemicals
Onion Bulb - 21 chemicals
Tomato Fruit - 21 chemicals
Oregano Plant - 21 chemicals
Soybean Seed - 19 chemicals
Black Currant Fruit - 19 chemicals
Tea Leaf - 18 chemicals
Rosemary Plant - 18 chemicals
Grape Fruit - 18 chemicals
Thyme Plant - 17 chemicals
Garlic Bulb - 16 chemicals
Cauliflower Leaf - 16 chemicals
Ginseng Plant - 16 chemicals
Paprika Fruit - 15 chemicals
Grapefruit Fruit - 15 chemicals
Sage Plant - 15 chemicals
Yarrow Plant - 14 chemicals
Tarragon Plant - 14 chemicals
Chili Fruit - 14 chemicals

(Dr. Duke's *Phytochemical and Ethnobotanical Database*, 1998)

Your body knows what those bad foods are; fried foods, fast foods, packaged foods, processed foods, sweets, pastries, baked goods, soda, fatty or greasy meats, cooked dairy products and high carb grains. Foods that make you tired, or swollen, or bloated, or grumpy. Foods that give you diarrhea, or constipate you, or stuff up your head and nose.

Anti-angiogenic Foods

Anti-angiogenic foods not only prevent cancer from occurring, they also prevent cancer activity; including limiting blood vessel growth to tumors and stopping cancer cells from metastasizing or spreading to other parts of your body (The Angiogenesis Foundation, 2010).

The Eat To Defeat Cancer Campaign is an excellent resource for information about foods with natural chemicals that fight against cancer. Read summaries of up to date studies like how eating tomato paste twice per week, lowered the risk of prostate cancer by 33% in 'Regular Consumption of Tomato Products Lowers Risk of Prostate Cancer' (The Angiogenesis Foundation, 2010). Here: www.eattodefeat.org

Search food by Fruits, Vegetables, Herbs & Spices, Seafood, Oils, Legumes, Grains & Seeds & Flours in, 'Here's The Evidence, News Supporting the Eat to Defeat Cancer Campaign' (The Angiogenesis Foundation, 2010). Here: www.eattodefeat.org

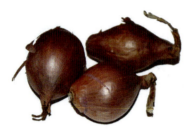

Apart from Red Clover, other known food plants with anti-angiogenic properties include green tea, dark chocolate and mineral rich maple syrup; several mushrooms including enoki, maitaki, reishi, shitake; herbs and spices including basil, black pepper, cinnamon, garlic, ginger, ginseng, licorice root, nutmeg, oregano, rosemary, tarragon and turmeric; fruits including apples, berries, all citrus, red grapes, pomegranate, peaches, cherries and cranberries; almost all vegetables, nuts and seeds including flax seed, sesame seed, cashews, pine nuts, chestnuts and walnuts; seaweeds including arame, dulse, kombu, mozuku, nori and wakame; and legumes including lentils, lima beans, soybeans, tofu and tempeh. To access the entire list go to Eat To Defeat Cancer (The Angiogenesis Foundation, 2010). Here: www.eattodefeat.org

In the video, *'Can we eat to starve cancer?'* on *Ted, Ideas Word Spreading*, Dr. William Li teaches about Angiogenesis and which foods we can eat to starve cancer (Li, 2010). Here: www.ted.com/talks/william_li.html

Abnormal angiogenesis is a hallmark of every type of cancer.

Dr. William Li, 2010.

Now, you are using your *power* and truly know you are a healing machine, have added *cleansing* to your arsenal, and are eating delicious, nutritious whole foods. Time to add another secret weapon – herbal medicine! Let's keep moving forward ... to Principle 4.

39   Principle 4 ~ Befriend Herbs!

Throughout this book you have learned the history of the use of herbs in natural medicine and their essential and important contributions to healing cancer. Here is a summary of the herbal preparations mentioned in this book, as well as a few more you may use to heal yourself.

Green Tea
Green tea is rich in flavonoids that fight cancer and anti-angiogenesis factors that inhibit metastases and blood vessel growth to tumors. Drink one or two cups every day. Green tea does contain caffeine and can cause symptoms of overstimulation such as heart palpitations and nervousness if taken in excess. It this happens, drink less, mix with water or substitute other less stimulating teas.

Turmeric Tea
Turmeric is the powdered root of the Curcuma Longa L. It is known in Ayurvedic medicine to be a *body cleanser*. It is a powerful antioxidant and is used to treat cancer in India. Turmeric has powerful anti-angiogenesis factors. One pinch in a cup, add boiling water, stir and enjoy as often as you like. Add a pinch to Chai tea, it has a mild, delicate flavor. Sprinkle in soups and add to rice, egg, grain or potato dishes often.

Your Own Healing Teas
Use the information in this book and in herbal books (there are several excellent books accessible through the Resource Section), to blend your own healing teas. Add a little Licorice root to balance out your blend. Add an herb that is slightly laxative and cleansing like Burdock, and one that is soothing and healing like Slippery Elm, Ginger or Lavender.

Bitter Tonic Tea™
All the herbs in Bitter Tonic Tea™ work together to kill pathogens like fungi, viruses and bacteria. They inhibit cancer growth, detoxify your body, cleanse out waste, boost your immune system and provide an abundance of minerals to rebalance the pH of your body's living fluids and nourish and protect your trillions of cells. The tea is gently expectorant and mildly laxative – expelling anything that does not belong.

Essiac™ Tea
Essiac tea has been used by thousands of people with much success, and many, many complete cures, over several decades. Put simply, the herbs

in Essiac work to kill cancer. Buy from an herbalist or health food store or make your own. A similar recipe is in Chapter 14 of this book.

Harry Hoxsey's Tea

There are many versions of his original tea on the internet and in books. The recipe for Bitter Tonic Tea above originated from Hoxsey's recipe. From his 1957 book, *You Don't Have To Die*, Harry tells us,

It stimulates the elimination of toxins which are poisoning the system, thereby corrects the abnormal blood chemistry and normalizes cell metabolism. Its ingredients are not secret. It contains potassium iodide combined with some or all of the following inorganic substances, as the individual case may demand: licorice, red clover, burdock root, stillingia root, barberis root, poke root, cascara, Aromatic USP 14, prickly ash bark, buckthorn bark . . . We prescribe the above medication in all cases of cancer, internal and external . . .

Harry Hoxsey in the 1957 book *You Don't Have To Die.*

Topical Herbal Compress

Any herb can be pulverized and mixed into a paste with water or food oil, like olive, sweet almond or sesame oil. Healing properties are absorbed through your skin and penetrate into the sub dermal layer beneath.

An alternative method, which is a little *less* messy, but just as effective is to make a very strong tea, soak a cotton ball, and tape it to the affected area.

Try any of the following herbs alone, or in combination, with a ratio of one part of each herb, for example 1 tablespoon of burdock root and 1 tablespoon of bloodroot.

Burdock Root
Chaparral Leaf
Bloodroot
Pau D'Arco

Cascara Sagrada
Astragalus
Red Clover Flowers
Golden Seal
Honeysuckle Flowers
Forsythia Flowers
Yellow Dock Root
Licorice

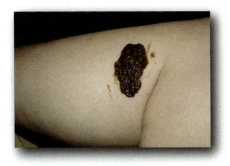

Medicinal Simple Teas

There are many herbs which work effectively to kill cancer and
regenerate your body when used alone. They can also be combined with
any other herbs listed here.

Use one or two teaspoons of dried herb for one cup of tea.

Red Clover Flowers
Burdock Root Tea
Burdock Leaf Tea
Pau D'Arco
Astragalus
Golden Seal
Sheep Sorrel
Licorice Root Tea
Sarsaparilla Root Tea
Oregon Grape Root
Dandelion Root Tea

Culinary Herbal Teas

Many of our wonderful culinary herbs also make effective cancer fighting
teas, by virtue of their high nutrient content and strongly scented oils
possessing potent anti-fungal properties. Try Rosemary, Oregano, Sage,
Thyme, Basil, Savory, Coriander, Cinnamon, Cardamom, Ginger,
Peppermint, Spearmint, Mountain Mint, Lavender or Lemon Balm alone
or in combination.

I would like to reiterate an important point about recipes for herbal
cancer remedies. Many herbs have anti-cancer properties and there have
been countless recipes which people have claimed are the *original* and
only recipe. They claim this so you will buy their preparation and avoid
others.

The herbal information and recipes shared in this book have been proven
to work because people used them and became well. We do not need
double blind placebo controlled studies to prove they work. Years and
years of experience is proof enough.

I like to think that Harry Hoxsey and Rene Caisse felt a sense of relief when they shared their recipes with others, just like Greg Caton who publicly shared his methods for making escharotic preparations. They must have known the information about herbal medicine which they held so close, should never be lost because of its massive potential to save so many millions of lives.

Herbs are here for everyone to use and benefit from. Knowledge about them belongs to no one person or organization. I have gladly given away hundreds of recipes for Bitter Tonic Tea over the last several years. Herbs and knowledge of their properties and use belong to *everyone*.

Do not be afraid or put off with the idea of making your own teas, it is really very effortless. Start with a simple tea, made of one herb, Pau D'Arco, Red Clover or Burdock; then begin mixing two or more, and move on to make Bitter Tonic Tea and other more complex formulas once you are comfortable working with herbs.

QUICK CANCER FIGHTING BLEND RED CLOVER, BURDOCK, AND PAU D'ARCO

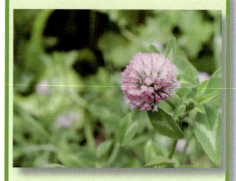

A quick cancer fighting herbal tea uses three of our strongest anti-cancer herbs, Red Clover, Burdock and Pau D'Arco, in equal quantities.

Use one teaspoon of each herb, pour boiled water over the herbs and let steep for at least 20 minutes or more. Drink 2 cups per day.

The point is to become friends with herbs so you know them intimately. They have properties and characteristics that can help you in many, many situations throughout your life. From the simple sedative qualities of lavender and chamomile tea for a stressed out headache to the more complex herbal blends which are rich with anti-cancer compounds, herbs are here to help and heal us. They are our friends! Why have we been ignoring them for so long? It is time to start a new friendship!

The next principle is crucial – getting rid of acid and rebalancing your pH.

40   Principle 5 ~ Get Rid Of Acid!

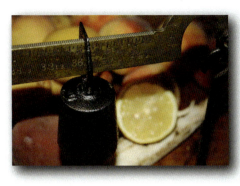

When my teenagers begin to feel the results of burning the candle at both ends and eating too much junk food they test their own pH. I smile to myself when they start making pH balancing green smoothies and salads, because I know they are learning to pay attention to signs their bodies are giving out. This helps them to manage their own eating patterns and take control of their health.

It is a simple but powerful strategy. Seeing the results of your recent bad food choices on a pH strip is a very motivating factor. You will see that choosing foods which nurture your body will make you feel better almost immediately. Retest, and you will see your pH is safely within the healthy range of 7.35 to 7.45.

Rebalancing pH is an integral part of natural cancer therapies. Cancer, aka fungus, grows in an acid and anaerobic or oxygen-less environment. Researchers have shown that malignant cells are acidic and healthy cells are alkaline. They believe that when the acidic pH of a cancer cell is changed to a more appropriate alkaline state, the body can repair the damaged DNA, reversing malignancy of the cancer cell!

Dr. Otto Heinrich Warburg, discovered the root cause of cancer in 1923 and was awarded a Nobel Prize in Physiology or Medicine for his discovery, *The Oxygen-Transferring Ferment of Respiration* (Warburg, 1931). Here: http://www.nobelprize.org/nobel_prizes/medicine/laureates/1931/warburg-lecture.html

What is pH anyway?
The literal meaning of pH is the potential of hydrogen. The potential of hydrogen to do what?

Hydrogen has the potential to react with other atoms by yielding or sharing its only electron. This forms a weak ionic bond, connecting the hydrogen atom to the atom receiving the electron. This bond is easily broken in solution, when mixed with another substance like water or blood for example.

Any substance that yields hydrogen ions in a solution is called an acid. The more hydrogen ions yielded, the stronger the acid. The stronger the acid, the more effective it is at breaking down substances. This is the essence of free radicals – unstable ions without one or more unpaired electrons. These highly reactive ions are deeply involved in degenerative diseases such as cancer, arthritis, osteoporosis, fibromyalgia and arterial disease.

Substances that accept or react with hydrogen ions are called bases. The more hydrogen ions accepted, the stronger the base or the more alkaline.

Our body uses bases to sop up acids and quell the damage they cause. These bases come from the alkaline minerals we take in with food or when necessary, pulled from the stores in our muscles, bones, teeth and organs.

The pH of our blood lies between 7.35 and 7.45, which makes it a weak basic solution. Our body prefers alkalinity. Acids make us sick and tired. They cause damage and inflammation to our tissues and cells and precipitate the release of essential minerals from stores throughout our body. Acids provide a fertile environment for yeasts and other pathogens and promote disease in our body.

The prime cause of the plague is the plague bacillus, but secondary causes of the plague are filth, rats, and the fleas that transfer the plague bacillus from rats to man. By a prime cause of a disease I mean one that is found in every case of the disease.

Cancer, above all other diseases, has countless secondary causes. But, even for cancer, there is only one prime cause. Summarized in a few words, the prime cause of cancer is the replacement of the respiration of oxygen in normal body cells by a fermentation of sugar.

All normal body cells meet their energy needs by respiration of oxygen, whereas cancer cells meet their energy needs in great part by fermentation. All normal body cells are thus obligate aerobes, whereas all cancer cells are partial anaerobes.

From the standpoint of the physics and chemistry of life this difference between normal and cancer cells is so great that one can scarcely picture a greater difference.

99

Dr. Otto Heinrich Warburg, 1969.

What causes overacidity to result?
Mild chronic acidosis often results from overconsumption of acid producing foods such as refined carbohydrates, damaged fats, sweets, alcohol, coffee, soda, meats and dairy products. Tobacco will also contribute to acidity in your body, as will prescription and recreational drugs, high stress levels, and low oxygen intake.

To reduce pH and eliminate acids from your body, eat less acid causing foods and more mineral rich green leafy vegetables, sea vegetables and fruits.

Fruits and vegetables with natural acids do not result in making our body and tissues more acidic. These acids, such as ascorbic acid or Vitamin C are used in many different processes throughout our body, leaving alkaline minerals behind for absorption and utilization. Although lemon juice has a pH of only 2.0, making it a strong acid, it produces alkalinity through releasing its mineral store, rather than producing acid residue and waste like damaged fat molecules, denatured proteins or psychotropic drugs, which over time can literally suck the minerals out of your bones and teeth, causing dangerous problems and chronic illness.

A less known cause of high acid levels is liver and gall bladder congestion. When alkaline bile cannot be properly expelled from the gall bladder because of a buildup of cholesterol, bile salts, toxins and fats, acidic chyme (food and stomach acid) continues down the digestive tract without being properly mixed with alkaline bile. This causes poor digestion, inferior assimilation of nutrients, heartburn, acid reflux, and damage to the small and large intestines, resulting in pain, discomfort, an aversion to many foods, lethargy and irritability.

How do you know if your pH is out of balance?
Your body has natural buffer systems that strive to keep your pH level in the safe range. A constant intake of acid producing foods causes these natural systems to become overworked and buffering substances begin to run out. Now your body begins to break down your muscles for alkalizing

glutamine and starts to heist alkalizing minerals like calcium, magnesium and potassium from your bones, teeth and organs.

When acid levels rise, fermentation takes place, causing oxygen levels within cells to decrease. Improper fat metabolism, caused by the intake of too many processed fats and not enough highly unsaturated fats, clogs cell membranes which also has an effect on the amount of oxygen within each cell, by causing cell wall permeability issues. This means nutrients cannot enter the cell properly and wastes cannot exit properly so accumulate inside the cell.

Mild chronic acidosis manifests in symptoms such as inflammation, dry skin, bleeding gums, brittle nails, thinning hair, irritability, fatigue, energy loss, joint pain and weakness, decreased immunity, yeast infections, kidney stones, digestive disturbances, colitis, Crohn's disease, acid reflux, indigestion, gall bladder and liver congestion and arterial damage (Brown and Trivieri, 2006).

Pay attention to symptoms from your body. These are important messages from the realm of true healing. If you do not *feeeeel* your normal self and suffer from one or more of the symptoms above, test your pH to be sure, but it will not hurt to add more alkaline foods anyway!

Once you become familiar with how poor you feel when your pH is on the acid side, and how lively and energetic you feel when your pH is more alkaline, you will come to know your pH without testing. For more information on how to test your pH, go to 'How To Test My Own pH.' Here: www.thegoodwitch.ca/how-to-test-my-own-ph/

How can I raise my pH to a more alkaline state?

In *The Acid Alkaline Food Guide*, the authors recommend an eating plan with 20% to 40% acid producing dairy, meat, fish and poultry and 60% to 80% alkaline producing fruits, vegetables, seeds, herbs and spices, with an emphasis on extremely alkalizing green leafy vegetables and root crops like burdock, radishes, turnips, carrots and parsnips (Brown & Trivieri, 2006).

When making changes to your diet, the most important thing is to focus on what you are putting in your body and how you *feeeeel* – before you eliminate or change anything! Make mental notes of any symptoms like joint pain or fatigue. Then after one or two days of really paying attention to what you are eating and how you *feeeeel*, begin nurturing and healing yourself by adding more alkaline, fresh, raw foods from the right side of the chart.

As you find foods and meals that suit your tastes, begin eliminating the foods that don't serve you anymore, from the left side of the chart. Making positive changes to your diet takes time but as you begin to *feeeel* the results, you will be motivated to continue.

Drinking plenty of fresh non-chlorinated water helps your kidneys flush excess acids. To improve alkalinity further, drink lemon water on waking every day. Fresh, raw lemon juice makes a delicious, refreshing, cleansing and alkaline drink when paired with strongly alkaline mineral water. Use the juice of half

PH SCALE OF COMMON FOODS

pH Scale of Common Foods

Download *pH Scale of Common Foods*. Print it out and tape it to your refrigerator. Make it larger on a photocopier if necessary. Focus on the foods on the right side of the scale. These are the foods that will sop up acids in your body with their rich reservoir of alkaline minerals. They will give you energy, oxygen and nutrients. Then you, as well as each one of your trillions of cells, will start to feel better as you become cleansed, nourished and protected.
Here: www.thegoodwitch.ca/ph-chart/

a lemon to a large glass of water. Brown and Trivieri tested hundreds of foods and beverages and recorded their results in *The Acid Alkaline Food Guide*. Here: www.thegoodwitch.ca/bookshelf/

They found of bottled mineral waters, the most alkaline were Apollinaris, San Pellegrino and Sanfaustino (Brown & Trivieri, 2006).

You *believe* you are healing, you use cleanses whenever needed, are eating superfoods every day, have herbal medicine on your side and now you need a little extra help deciding which supplements to take.

Next . . . Natural Supplementation!

41 Principle 6 ~ Natural Supplementation!

Supplementation is meant to cover any nutritional shortcomings in the food we eat. If we are short on iron, wouldn't it make perfect sense to just eat some more iron rich foods like sun-dried iron rich apricots? When a craving for chocolate is caused by a deficiency in magnesium, does it not make sense to satisfy your craving by eating delicious, high quality, eco and people friendly dark chocolate?

Cravings serve a purpose, they are messages from your body, and should never be ignored! Cravings for food or sweets in particular can be caused by yeast imbalance or broad spread nutritional deficiencies.

The closer you eat to Principle 3 ~ Super Nutrition, the faster your body will build its stores of all nutrients, and the less deficiencies and cravings you will experience. For example, fast food doesn't fill a need for nutrients, it fills a need for mass, or calories. If you eat a big juicy burger, you'll be hungry shortly after because your body couldn't find the nutrients it was craving. Unless you choose to put nutrients into your body, your body will keep craving *stuff*. Your body craves nutrients, not calories.

Immune Boosting, Cancer Fighting, Garlic and Onions

Garlic and onions inherently carry powerful cancer fighting chemicals. Why wouldn't we use them?

Thousands of studies have proven the anti-carcinogenic properties of raw garlic and onions. Fresh garlic and aged garlic extract in particular are highly effective at inhibiting the growth of cancer.

A review of the literature in *Journal of Nutrition*, 'Enhanced Immunocompetence by Garlic: Role in Bladder Cancer and Other Malignancies,' shows that garlic has strong inhibitory action against the growth of cancer. Garlic is directly toxic to gastric, colon, bladder and prostate cancer and to sarcomas, cancers arising in muscle, bone, bladder, kidneys, liver, lungs, parotid glands (behind the ear) and spleen (Lamm, 2001).

The studies reviewed, show garlic detoxifies carcinogens by stimulating enzymes, antioxidants and sulfur, to bind to and remove them. It stimulates lymphocytes (immune cells) to proliferate, increases phagocytosis (engulfing and destroying microorganisms) by macrophages, encourages macrophages and lymphocytes to attack transplanted tumors in animals, enhances activity of natural killer cells, killer cells and lymphokine-activated killer cells. Garlic stimulates the release of cytokines or immune regulators, interleukin-2, tumor necrosis factor and interferon. The components of garlic regulate and enhance the process of the immune response, and the activity of immune cells and organs. Garlic maintains stimulation of the immune system as long as it is added to your diet on a regular basis, which can significantly reduce the incidence of cancer (Lamm, 2001).

Garlic is mentioned in the oldest known medical text on earth, from 1550 BCE, the *Egyptian Ebers Papyrus*. Garlic was reportedly fed to Egyptian soldiers to maintain their strength and vitality, and has been used by every civilization on earth (Bowden, 2007).

Among garlic's multitude of virtues are its potent anti-cancer properties. Study after study shows garlic extract effective at reducing cancer risk, having chemopreventive effects, suppressing cancer cell proliferation, promoting apoptosis or programmed cell death, and having powerful cancer fighting abilities, to kill cancer cells, prevent tumor growth, and inhibit metastases.

One evening, while my mother lay dying in palliative care, I decided to stop for a bottle of wine. I had been crying on the way there and a woman who was offering samples of wine instantly noticed something was wrong. She asked me if I was okay, so I told her my mother was dying. She told me a story about her friend who cured herself with aged garlic extract, known as Kyolic garlic. She said her friend took Kyolic regularly, and claimed it was the only therapy she used!

Garlic is an amazing herbal therapy. The most perfect example of medicinal food, it has been used for everything from the common cold to leprosy and cancer!

Why would raw garlic and onions be effective against cancer cells? They are both rich in immune boosting nutrients like selenium, sulphur and trace minerals, but their real power lies in antifungal, anti-viral, antibacterial and anti-parasitic properties. Garlic kills pathogens, and is particularly good at killing fungal cells, hence it's ability to inhibit the proliferation of many different kinds of cancer cells.

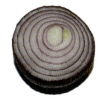

A search for garlic on Dr. Duke's *Phytochemical and Ethnobotanical Database,* brings back a massive list of natural chemicals in garlic with anti-cancer properties, including immune modulators, antileukemic, antilymphomic, antimutagenic, anti proliferant, antistaphylococcic, anti-tumor, anti-tumor (colon), antiviral, candidicide, fungicide, cancer-preventive, antibacterial, amebicide, immunostimulant, insecticide, larvicide, mycobactericide, nematicide, phagocytotic, antibiotic, hepatoprotective, anti-cancer, chemopreventive, anti-cancer (stomach), anti-tumor (stomach), anti-tumor (bladder) and anti-tumor (prostate) (Dr. Duke's *Phytochemical and Ethnobotanical Database*, 1998).

The properties above are from the chemicals in garlic that start with 'A' only! Some you may recognize, some you may not: Adenosine, Diallyl Sulfide, Ajoene, Alanine, Allicin, Alliin, Allixin, Allyl-Methyl-Disulfide, Allyl-Methyl-Trisulfide, Alpha Phellandrene, Alpha-tocopherol, Arachidonic-acid, Ascorbic Acid (Dr. Duke's *Phytochemical and Ethnobotanical Database*, 1998).

To search the database yourself, go to Dr. Duke's *Phytochemical and Ethnobotanical Database*, type 'garlic' in the search bar, click submit query, highlight 'garlic' and click the radio box 'Print activities with chemicals', then click submit query again. Voila – garlic's list of chemicals and all their health giving properties. Here: www.ars-grin.gov/duke/plants.html

Fresh raw garlic chopped small and taken on a spoon with water . . . Fresh raw garlic, dehydrated garlic, garlic powder and onions added to salads, sandwiches, rice or potato dishes . . . *Heavenly Garlicky Hummus*, Aged garlic extract . . .   Allicin rich garlic pills . . . it really does not matter which way you take it, as long as it is in a raw or dehydrated state, all nutrients will be present and available to you. Just get it in you! Here: www.thegoodwitch.ca/heavenly-garlicky-hummus/

Immune Boosting Selenium

Selenium is an essential trace element directly involved in immune protection. It is a potent cancer fighter and low intakes of this important nutrient are associated with increased rates of many different cancers.

Selenium functions as an antioxidant, and is considered up to five hundred times more potent than Vitamin E, which it works alongside. Selenium is known for improving longevity, immune stimulation, removing mercury buildup and normalizing blood pressure.

The best source of selenium is fresh raw nuts, in particular brazil nuts. Selenium is also found in garlic, onions, broccoli, tomatoes, brown rice, wheat germ, sunflower seeds, cashews, wild fish, eggs and whole grains, all foods you will eat more of when you follow Principle 3 ~ Super Nutrition.

Culinary Herbs

The aromatic oils of culinary herbs like Parsley, Dill, Rosemary, Thyme, Oregano, Sage and Basil have potent anti-fungal and anti-cancer properties.

Culinary herbs are also rich in vitamins, minerals and phytochemicals and add a whole new dimension of flavor and nutrition to your meals. Fresh, dark green herbs are also an excellent source of chlorophyll, which purifies your blood, kills pathogens and nourishes your tissues and organs.

The umbelliferous vegetables, including parsley, fennel and dill carry a cancer fighting volatile oil called Myristicin. Myristicin stimulates the production of glutathione, an important detoxifying enzyme produced in your liver, spleen, small intestinal lining, and within all cells, which acts as their personal immune system.

This puts Parsley among a special group of foods with the highest anti-cancer activity of all (Bowden, 2007).

Culinary herbs are always better fresh, but in winter months, dried herbs are an excellent substitute. Culinary herbs also make heavenly teas. Iced teas made from fruit teas and herbs make refreshing and nutritious summer drinks.

GROWING ROSEMARY

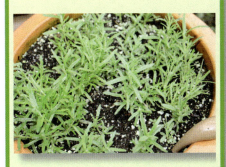

One package of Rosemary seeds spreads nicely over a large pot.

These midsummer plants will yield enough Rosemary for the entire winter for our family, for fragrant Rosemary tea, to add to potato and vegetable dishes, or to mix in herbal blends like Italian seasoning, for dips, breads, salads, soups and casseroles.

Rosemary also makes a comforting winter tea.

Rosemary is a tender perennial and must be grown inside during winter in northern climates. It is difficult to re-climatize indoors and the plants don't recover well after harvesting, so they are composted.

As with medicinal herbs, growing culinary herbs in your own organic garden is the best way to become familiar with their qualities and benefits and comfortable with your favorite ways to use them.

Make your own herbal seasoning blend with herbs grown in your garden or purchased from your local farmers' market. Make Italian seasoning with: Oregano, Basil, Parsley, Thyme, Garlic and Rosemary. Make

Stuffing (poultry) seasoning with: Thyme, Rosemary, Sage, Parsley, Savory and Onion powder.

Don't be shy with culinary herbs. Chop them into green or pasta salads, layer them in sandwiches, or roll them up and cut into thin ribbons to sprinkle on soups or roll into Japanese maki.

Use them alone or mix them together. There is nothing more delicious than chopped fresh rosemary and basil on salads in the summer, fresh from the garden.

A few years ago I planted one seed package of thyme in my organic vegetable garden. Now I have a patch of Thyme that provides our family with fresh Thyme all summer and dried thyme during winter months for teas and herbal blends.

Mix together dried herbs such as Oregano, Thyme, Basil and Rosemary, store in a glass jar and use all winter to sprinkle in soups, salads, casseroles and baked potatoes or mix into carrot and sweet potato mash along with a blob of organic butter and a sprinkling of unrefined, mineral rich sea salt.

Immune Enhancing Mushrooms

Thousands of studies show the immune modulating and anti-tumor benefits of mushrooms. In particular, Maitake, Reishi and Shitake mushrooms improve immune function. They help to increase the activity of natural killer cells and other immune cells. Make them a regular part of your diet.

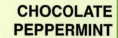

CHOCOLATE PEPPERMINT

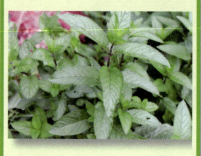

Chocolate Peppermint ready for harvest

Peppermint contains many anti-cancer properties including alpha-carotene, alpha-pinene, alpha-terpineol, alpha-tocopherol, beta-carotene, beta-ionone, chlorogenic-acid, and many, many more.

During summer months add chocolate mint leaves to raspberry iced tea. Use two raspberry tea bags, and chopped mint leaves, pour boiling water over them and let steep for at least ten minutes. Let cool or add ice if you are in a hurry. Squeeze in the juice of half to one lemon, add stevia, raw agave nectar or unpasteurized honey to taste.

Most supermarkets and health food stores carry several varieties of mushrooms in fresh or dried forms. Buy the whole fresh mushrooms and slice into salads or onto sandwiches. Dehydrated mushrooms can be refreshed in a little water, then sliced and added to soups, salads, casseroles or sandwiches.

Dried medicinal mushrooms like Shitake can be made into a tea, by crushing them in a mortar and pestle and pouring boiling water over them. Let steep at least twenty minutes.

Laetrile or B17

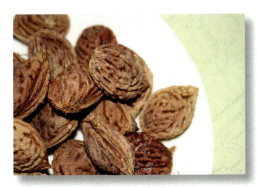

Do you remember the Hunzakuts from Hunza?

They are one group of centenarians who live in excellent health until their death, usually over the age of 100!

One of the secrets of the Hunzakuts is they grow organic apricots, which are sun dried on the roofs of their homes. In fact, in Hunza a person's wealth is measured by the number of apricot trees SHe owns!

What is so important about the apricots? Apart from being an incredibly nutritious and alkalizing food, rich in protective antioxidants and cancer fighting carotenes, the apricots hold a tiny powerhouse of cancer fighting B17 in their seeds! To the Hunzakuts, even more prized than the apricot itself, is the tiny bitter seed inside. The Hunzakuts eat as many apricot seeds as they do apricots! (Griffin, 1974).

According to G. Edward Griffin, in the documentary, *A World Without Cancer*, "there has never been a reported case of cancer among the Hunzakuts." This movie focuses on the benefits of B17 and suggests that we are more susceptible to cancer when deficient in B17, which is considered to be an essential nutrient of a healthy diet.

A natural diet with emphasis on plant foods, like that of the Hunzakuts and other centenarians, will provide not only B17, but many other cancer preventive nutrients as well (Griffin, 1974).

B17 or Laetrile is component of the tiny bitter seed found inside the hard pit of *drupe* fruits like apricot, peach, nectarine and plum. It is also found in sufficient quantities inside tiny apple seeds. I learned many years ago from a farmer friend that horses naturally deworm themselves in the fall by eating copious amounts of apples and their tiny *poisonous* seeds!

Laetrile is a controversial compound because it is a complex molecule that includes toxic cyanide. However as Griffin shows in *A World*

184

Without Cancer, in small quantities, like those found naturally in drupe fruit seeds, cyanide is very effective at killing cancer cells without hurting you! (Griffin, 1974).

Apricot seeds are characteristic in their medicinal similarity to herbs; that of being very helpful in small doses and harmful in large quantities.

We have thrown away knowledge of our natural medicines and their benefits, but we have also thrown out the medicines themselves! If we were living in tune with nature, we would eat several dozen drupe fruits each summer season, and nature would expect that we would eat the seeds. However, we have given up eating these seeds and throw them out with the pit.

Now the tiny cancer fighting drupe fruit seeds can be purchased at your local health food store. This is the best form of course, the fresh seed itself, not the seed dehydrated, ground and stuffed into a glycerin shell, waiting on a shelf for months . . .

Vitamin and Mineral Supplements

Many vitamin and mineral supplements on the market are synthetic, processed and bound with fillers. Instead, look for natural, whole-food, *green* supplements made from a base of sea vegetables and whole, ground up plants. Seaweeds are a powerhouse of proteins, phytochemicals, vitamins, minerals, essential fats, and trace elements. They nourish and support all systems of your body. Your green supplement should also contain a variety of raw berries, fruits, vegetables, herbs, spices, seeds and nuts to provide the richest and most bio-available source of nutrients. These natural formulas come in powder or liquid form. Your health food store can lead you to the healthiest and most effective, natural, whole foods and green supplements; or go to www.thegoodwitch.ca/cauldron_shop/ for our most trusted suppliers.

Raw, Organic Whey Protein Isolate

Immunocal™ is a very high quality form of protein and in particular it is rich in cysteine, a precursor amino acid for the production of glutathione. A precursor is a raw material used to produce something, which simply means without cysteine your cells cannot make glutathione. Glutathione is a tripeptide molecule, made of cysteine, glutamic acid and glycine, three amino acids of the twenty-two which comprise the building blocks of all known proteins (Somersall & Bounous, 2001).

Glutathione is your body's premier biochemical antioxidant. Present in all cells, it plays a critical role in cell-defense. Your glutathione antioxidant system is the way your cells protect themselves, their own tiny immune system. Glutathione destroys reactive oxygen compounds, those nasty free radicals that bounce around damaging critical DNA structures, and causing mutations. It also plays a key role in defending your body against infections by bacteria, viruses and fungi and protects cells against the damaging effects from foreign chemicals, pollutants and xenobiotics (Somersall & Bounous, 2001).

Normal levels of glutathione inside your spleen and immune cells are essential for the continuous multiplication of lymphocytes and the production of antibodies. Glutathione maintains other antioxidants such as Vitamin C and E, to protect your body against disease.

Studies show that glutathione levels in the body do not increase when it is taken in oral supplement form (Somersall & Bounous, 2001).

This vast body of research shows that glutathione interrupts common mechanisms that both destroy cells and cause many types of degenerative disease.

Somersall & Bounous, 2001.

Immunotec holds several Canadian, U.S. and International patents for its immune enhancing products, including U.S. Patent 5,230,902, July 27, 1993, 'Undenatured Whey Protein Concentrate to improve active systemic humoral immune response;' and Australian Patent 46937-93, January 19, 1995, 'Anti-Cancer Therapeutic Composition containing whey protein concentrate' (Immunotec, 2010).

What is so special about Immunocal™?

Why don't other whey protein isolates have the same effect on cancer?

Immunocal™ is made from raw cow's milk, but it is the patented process used by Immunotec which preserves all nutrients, including the delicate amino acid cysteine, which your body uses to make protective glutathione.

The humoral (mediated by B cells, a bodily defense reaction that recognizes virus, fungi, or bacteria and produces specific antibodies against them) immune response in mice fed raw whey protein was almost 500% higher than mice fed a casein diet, even when the casein diet was enriched with cysteine! The raw whey protein was the key. Some cases improved the life span of mice by thirty percent! (Somersall & Bounous, 2001).

186

As I dissected the animals that morning, I was blown away. The results absolutely stunned me. Livers of the first two groups of mice were spotted with gray, cancerous tumors, but the big surprise was the whey-fed group's livers. They remained completely unspotted . . . they were pink . . . and obviously normal. Colon tumors were significantly less too.

Somersall and Bounous, 2001.

To find more information regarding Immunotec the company, Immunocal™ the raw isolated whey protein supplement, or the man Dr. Gustavo Bounous and his extensive research with immune enhancing products at the world renowned McGill University in Montreal, Canada. See the Resources section at the back of this book.

For more information about Immunocal, the immune enhancing product. Here: www.thegoodwitch.ca/cauldron_shop/

It was demonstrated that this immune enhancing activity of the whey protein concentrate was related to greater production of splenic glutathione during oxygen-requiring, antigen-driven clonal expansion of the lymphocyte pool. In addition, mice fed the whey protein concentrate exhibited higher levels of tissue glutathione which was believed to account for observed anti-tumor effects and even favorable effects on natural aging.

Somersall & Bounous, 2001

Note: Isolated Whey Protein is a high quality protein source, and is not considered a major source of calcium.

Dr. Bounous' discovery sounds very similar to Johanna Budwig's cottage cheese protocol, minus the immune boosting flax oil.

Both therapies use high quality protein in its most active form that is not denatured by the pasteurization process, to provide the body with amino acids, the precursor raw materials for the production of glutathione and other active components of the immune system.

Even today, medicine still has not widely accepted the fact that nutrition undeniably plays an enormous role in both prevention and treatment of major diseases.

Dr. Gustavo Bounous, 2001.

Harold Jansma tells how the active proteins in Immunocal helped his body to heal itself:

In June 1999, at age 40, I was diagnosed with a large tumour wrapped around the pineal gland in my brain. When first scanned it was 3.2 cm and growing rapidly.

Surgery was a very risky option. Chemotherapy was recommended. The oncologist suggested I probably had up to 12 weeks to live, possibly 6 to 12 months at the outside.

In one week's time, additional testing showed the tumour had grown to 3.8 cm.

I remember how much my dad suffered undergoing standard medical treatments for cancer. With my wife's agreement and support, I decided to forego the medical treatments.

We spent a few days researching non-stop. The one thing we found that seemed most relevant was the need for glutathione. By chance, at a recent doctor's appointment, I had picked up an Immunocal brochure that was slipped into a magazine in the MD's waiting room. I suddenly remembered it, because I remembered reading about glutathione in that brochure.

I ordered Immunocal and started taking 4 packets per day. One week later I increased to 6 per day, as recommended by my Immunotec consultant. I continued at 6 packets per day into July, and continue to feel better all the time. In late July my new MRI showed significant reduction in the tumour size. My MD agreed it made sense for me to continue what I was doing, and not do the standard chemo treatments.

99

Harold Jansma, Burstall, Saskatoon, Canada.

In April 2010, over ten years later, Harold continues to enjoy good health. The only intervention he used to regain his health was high doses of Immunocal (Connie McCracken, Immunotec Consultant, 2010).

Now that you are supplementing with whole, natural, power packed, nutritious foods, it is time to breathe deeply and add movement to your cancer fighting repertoire . . .

42 Principle 7 ~ Move and Breathe!

John Robbins discusses the daily activity built into the lives of centenarians, "Retirement is an unknown concept in Abkhasian thinking. The Abkhasians never, at any stage of life, become sedentary. Most of the elderly still work regularly, many in the orchards and gardens, pruning the fruit and nut trees, removing dead wood, and planting young trees. Some still chop wood and haul water" (Robbins, 2006).

Constant activity in daily life of the Abkhasians develops the function of their heart and lungs to a large degree, increasing the amount of oxygen supplied to their hearts, organs and cells (Robbins, 2006).

Moving your body helps lymph fluids circulate. Your lymphatic system does not have a pumping system like your cardiovascular system. Instead it relies on the movement of your large muscles and bones to push and squeeze lymph fluid through its venous tubes and disease fighting nodes. You must move to heal your body, but it does not have to be uncomfortable or boring!

What movement is the best and most effective?

One that you love doing!

There are so many ways to move your body and an infinite number of places to do it.

Try a variety of activities until you find a combination that keeps you fit and happy.

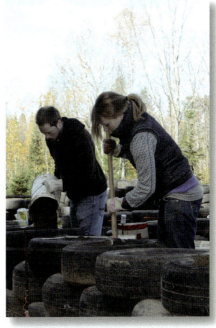

Alix & Stefan getting a workout and lots of fresh air, pounding tires for an Earth House!

Some activities that involve movement but do not feel like *exercise* include walking, hiking, competitive sports, gardening, sweeping,

190

vacuuming, raking, shoveling, dancing, swimming, going up and down stairs, playing, cleaning or working outside.

These activities also shape your body, burn fat, help to detoxify and move wastes through your body and improve the function of all your bodily systems, including your immune system.

Your needs for movement change constantly so be kind to yourself by paying attention to how you feel and move accordingly. If your energy levels are low maybe it is time to take a break and just do a sun salutation or rest, but if you are feeling extra energetic and want to play tennis after you just played a game of hockey or walked for three hours, go for it!

One type of *movement* that helps to break up pockets of congestion throughout your body is yoga. It gently and effectively stretches out ligaments, muscles, tissues and organs. Another is tai chi!

They make you *feeeeel* wonderful, strong and powerful. You will stand up straight and love the body you are in.

There are many different types of yoga, so you may have to try a few before you find one that resonates with you. I remember the very first class I ever tried, I fell asleep and that really was not the type of yoga I was looking for! I was disillusioned for a while until I tried another instructor who taught more powerful, fluid movement, and now I absolutely love my yoga class!

You do not have to go to classes, although having the benefit of a knowledgeable instructor can be very helpful. Yoga and Tai Chi DVD's and books are available everywhere and free videos and instructions are available on the web.

Another extremely useful and simple exercise is walking. Walking is the easiest exercise and requires almost no equipment; you can walk anywhere, anytime with proper clothing. You only need a pair of running shoes or comfortable walking shoes and if you happen to feel like stepping it up a notch after a few walks, throw a little jog or run in there, or hike through a forest or field. The more you move, the more you will want to move, the easier it will become, and the stronger you will feel . . . and be!

Movement increases breath. This is important for many reasons, including increasing oxygen levels throughout your body. Cancer cells require an anaerobic or oxygen-less environment and *cannot* live and thrive in a oxygenated environment. Movement also stimulates the removal of toxins from your lungs through deep breathing and oxygen helps to alkalize your blood and tissues. So breathe and breathe deeply!

Practice breathing with your stomach. While lying on your back, use your diaphragm to pull air into the bottom of your lungs. Your diaphragm is a muscle, which gets weak and small when you don't use it; use it and make it big and strong, so it is able to pull oxygen into your lungs quickly and efficiently. Push your stomach out while the bottom of your lungs fill with air. Then continue your in-breath, filling the top of your lungs, by expanding your chest. Now exhale, deflating the tops of your lungs by compressing your chest, then deflating the bottom of your lungs by compressing your stomach. Breathe all the air out of your lungs, sending the toxins with it.

When I first began to breathe properly again, after many years of not realizing I was using only shallow chest breathing, I literally had to force my stomach up and out to fill my lungs. Now my stomach moves naturally with breathing because my diaphragm is strong and effective. It took some time and effort to build my diaphragm up again. Just be persistent and always breathe deeply from your stomach first.

Be aware of compressing your breathing by slouching in your chair. Be conscious of sitting up straight to facilitate air flow in and out of your lungs. Practicing yoga or stretching and strengthening your core muscles on a regular basis will encourage your back to sit tall and straight, all of the time, without any conscious effort on your part.

Breath is also an ideal tool for reducing stress, something we will talk more about in Principle 9. But first, next up is Sunshine . . .

43 Principle 8 ~ Sunshine And Vitamin D!

Vitamin D develops from our interaction with our beautiful sun. We literally absorb the sun's energy and use it to keep ourselves alive! This hormone like vitamin is essential for a healthy body; without it we would die.

Vitamin D is *really* a hormone produced in your skin from absorption of sunlight, providing a necessary compound is available in the epidermal layer of your skin. The precursor sterol 7-dehydrocholesterol, a modified steroid hormone made from cholesterol, goes through several changes until Vitamin D3 is formed. Vitamin D3 is absorbed in your bloodstream and stored in fat in your liver (University of California, Riverside, 2000).

As needed, Vitamin D is released from the liver, and carried to the kidneys where it is converted to its active form. What does this hormone really do?

Vitamin D performs many important functions in your body, including modulating immune function and inhibiting the proliferation of cells by stimulating their differentiation or specialization. It assists in the metabolism of calcium and phosphorous into bones and teeth during bone growth and repair. Adequate levels of Vitamin D prevent rickets in children and osteoporosis in adults. Vitamin D deficiency symptoms can include insomnia, nearsightedness, psoriasis, burning in throat and mouth, muscle cramps, ticks and weakness, nosebleeds, racing heart, bone pain, malformation of bones and teeth, dental cavities, arthritis, osteomalacia, osteoporosis and rickets (Perrault, 2001).

According to a new study published in the March 2010 issue of the *Journal of Clinical Endocrinology and Metabolism*, an unbelievable fifty-nine percent of study subjects were Vitamin D deficient, with almost twenty-five percent showing extremely low levels of Vitamin D. The study also showed that the more people were deficient in Vitamin D, the more fat they carried! (McGill University Newsroom, 2010).

The study's principal investigator, Dr. Richard Kremer reports, 'Vitamin D insufficiency is a risk factor for other diseases . . . because it is linked to increased body fat, it may affect many different parts of the body. Abnormal levels of Vitamin D are associated with a whole spectrum of diseases, including cancer, osteoporosis and diabetes, as well as cardiovascular and autoimmune disorders' (McGill University Newsroom, 2010).

You can read more information about this important study in the McGill University newsroom, 'Low levels of Vitamin D linked to muscle fat, decreased strength in young people' (McGill University Newsroom, 2010). Here: http://www.mcgill.ca/newsroom/news/item/? item_id=115221

Vitamin D deficiency can be caused by inadequate sun exposure and excessive use of sunscreens. Do not use commercial sunscreens, as they contain toxic chemicals that are readily absorbed by your skin. Some of these chemicals increase your risk of skin cancer. There are many natural, non-harmful sunscreens available in natural health stores.

My family has never used sunscreen. When my children were small they were taught to throw on a T-shirt and hat or get out of the sun, if their skin was starting to burn. They have beautiful healthy tans every summer and an abundance of Vitamin D stored in their liver for the long, dark winter months ahead. We are not worried about skin cancer because our diet is full of protective, antioxidants and immune enhancing nutrients such as essential fats, minerals and vitamins C and A from fresh and raw fruits, herbs, vegetables, seeds, nuts, legumes and grains.

A more hidden cause of Vitamin D deficiency can be improper absorption or metabolism of Vitamin D due to intestinal disturbances such as Crohn's Disease or Colitis, or improper metabolism of fats and cholesterols caused by congestion in your gall bladder and liver. These may take the form of gallstones and fatty liver. Congestion in your liver and gallbladder can cause numerous identifying symptoms. For more information about this particular condition read, 'Conversations with Dr. Gall.' Here: www.thegoodwitch.ca/conversations-with-dr-gall/

If you want to skip this informative story because you know you require a Liver/Gall Bladder cleanse, enter your email at www.TheGoodWitch.ca for instant access to Cleanse Your Body!, with nine healing cleanses, including detailed instructions for the Liver/Gall Bladder cleanse. Here: www.thegoodwitch.ca/start-with-cleanses-first/

To increase your sun exposure, spend at least thirty minutes outside every day, whether the sun is shining or the clouds are showing. Combine sun exposure with a brisk walk and you have not only boosted your immune enhancing Vitamin D levels, you have stimulated your lymph system with movement; two great cancer fighters.

If you live in a northern climate you are more prone to developing cancer. Low light levels in winter translates to low Vitamin D levels in the body, so it is important to supplement if you are not outside regularly.

Taking Vitamin D capsules in the summer while exposing yourself to the sun can cause a dangerous buildup of Vitamin D in your liver.

Vitamin D supplements should only be taken during winter months when natural light levels are low.

Take Vitamin D_3 supplements in oil form, or in Cod Liver Oil or Halibut Oil or use the old fashioned winter remedy of hanging around outside to absorb sun energy through your eyes, face and hands . . . or you could take a vacation in the sunny south!

Some foods naturally contain Vitamin D and can be used to increase levels in the body if needed. The best sources include cod and halibut liver oils, and salmon, tuna and mackerel flesh. Small quantities of Vitamin D are in butter, cheese, eggs and yogurt (University of California, Riverside, 2000); keep in mind however that these foods contribute to congestion in your body if eaten in excess.

The next principle is one you will enjoy immensely – pampering yourself!

44 Principle 9 ~ Be Good To Yourself!

Slooooow Down, Relax and Rejuvenate.

There is a point to being alive, and it is not to suffer!

So, why do we stress ourselves out so much?

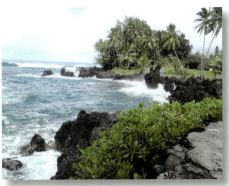

Simply placing focus on yourself, will give you the courage to say, 'No' when you need to, to take some time to relax every day, and to do the things you enjoy.

Take stock of your present situation. How do you spend your days? Is there something you could be doing that would help to relax and rejuvenate you?

Beautiful Maui Coast, Photo by Sue Witchel

Only you know what rejuvenates your body and soul. For some, it may be spending time with family and for others, it may be basking in the sun on a beautiful beach, planting tomatoes in the garden, or surfing the rugged volcanic coastline of Maui.

Spend at least one day of every week rejuvenating yourself. This will pay off in your business and family life and allow you to deal with stressful situations with compassion and understanding. One day a week, every week – for you . . .

Soak Up Negative Ions!

It is too bad negative ions are referred to as '*negative*' because they are so essential to good health. Humans and other animals absorb small ions, negative and positive. It is the balance of ions, or the electrical *soup* we live in that has enormous effects on our health. When ions are removed from the air over growing plants, their growth becomes stunted and plants become diseased. Conversely when ion levels are increased, plants flourish. As far back as 1748, L'Abbe Nollet placed plants under charged electrodes and found they grew faster. This electrical energy, created by friction in weather patterns and the sun's radiation, is all around us. Like fish in a sea of water, we live in a sea of electricity.

Too many pos-ions can bring ill health. From the Foehn of central Europe to the Sharav of the Middle East, as the wind falls and blows, it brings dry air and an abundance of positively charged ions (Soyka & Edmonds, 1977). Locals know the symptoms well, that come with the dry winds, feeling tense, anxious and depressed, in the days before the winds arrive.

In Geneva, my neighbor suffered from tension and anxiety during the Foehn in addition to migraine headaches. After several years of pill taking, she found her own solution to the most acute attacks. In the center of Geneva the lake narrows and flows over a small waterfall to become the River Rhone. At that point there is a bridge for pedestrians to cross the river. Each day during the Foehn she would spend between thirty minutes and an hour leaning over the railings, absorbed by the dancing waterfall and the swirl and eddy of the water. In fact she explained, "I go there just to breathe. It makes me feel better for hours.

Soyka & Edmonds, 1977

The friction in moving water creates neg-ions, which are abundant in the fine spray around waterfalls and in fresh, clean air of mountainous areas. Humans are naturally drawn to such places to rest and recuperate (Soyka & Edmonds, 1977). The creation of neg-ions by falling water explains why we feel so refreshed and energized after a shower, after a spring rain, near waterfalls, in the woods and mountains, and after a thunderstorm.

In 'Treatment of Seasonal Affective Disorder with a High-Output Negative Ionizer,' the authors conclude high-density negative ionizers can be used to treat seasonal affective disorder (Terman & Terman, 1995). Here: http://www.ncbi.nlm.nih.gov/pubmed/9395604

We know this illness well in the northern hemisphere during winter months. By late winter, the dry, pos-ion air has us wishing for sun, rain and the fresh electricity carried in with spring thunderstorms.

De-Stress

Stress is a barrier to happiness. It stagnates energy, causes illness and disease, creates anxiety and hampers creativity. Stress impedes personal and business relationships and reduces your quality of life. Many studies show that stress of any kind impedes healing; whether you are undergoing constant stress, such as providing ongoing care for a dying loved one, or temporary stress, such as that caused by preparing for a speech or school examination.

> **STRESSED? EXTEND YOUR OUT BREATH!**
>
> Take ten relaxing breaths. Inhale through your nose for a count of four, and exhale through your mouth for a count of eight. Slow your breath, close your eyes if possible, and relax. This technique automatically relaxes your nervous system, allowing you to calmly reenter an otherwise stressful situation, and handle it without agitation or anger. It can be done anywhere, anytime, in any situation! Ten breaths...

It is imperative then to reduce stress by making decisions about what influences you let into your life. Reduce unnecessary responsibilities, limit your exposure to media, remove yourself from stressful situations and stay away from negative people who create and focus on problems.

Do not waste time doing something unless it is what you truly want. Do what makes you happy; your life will be vibrant, successful and worth living.

Improve your ability to handle stress by meditating, replacing negative thoughts with opposite positive thoughts, doing yoga, getting close to nature, taking time for yourself, moving regularly, getting lots of restful sleep and practicing deep breathing.

Reducing your response to stressful situations can also help. Reacting more stressfully than needed can accelerate the situation and cause undue anxiety and worry. We have a large amount of control over our reaction to stressful situations. When you come across a stressful event, stop, take note of how you feeeel and do not let yourself get caught up in the situation. Breathe . . .

Rest and Sleep

Adequate sleep is imperative to your healing process. During sleep, your body is busy performing activities that detoxify, cleanse and rejuvenate your tissues and organs. Without proper rest, your body has a hard time keeping up with important cleansing activities.

Sleep on an empty stomach to facilitate your body's natural cleansing cycle.

Go to bed early enough to always get a good night's sleep. You want to feel refreshed on waking, not miserable and tired!

If you have trouble relaxing, herbal teas can be very helpful. Chamomile, Rosemary, Oat Straw and Lemon Balm are all calming teas. Lavender, although known mainly as a perfume scent, makes a wonderful calming tea. Try mixing herbs for a more complex flavor, Lavender and Chamomile or Rosemary and Lemon Balm, or blend all of the above herbs in equal parts.

Avoid drinks with caffeine, peppermint or licorice after 6:00 p.m., as they can be too stimulating and keep you awake at night.

Your body uses magnesium to relax your muscles. Tense up your fist . . . you are using calcium. Now relax it . . . you are using magnesium. Can you see how too much calcium and not enough magnesium can cause you to be too tight?

Without adequate amounts of magnesium you may experience muscle cramping and twitching, insomnia, irritability and the inability to relax. Soaking in a warm bath with a half cup of Epsom salts will increase your magnesium levels, help to relax your muscles and calm you before bed. Epsom salts are pure Magnesium Sulfate.

Make a soothing herbal sachet with Epsom Salts, Lavender, Chamomile, Rosemary, Oat Straw and Lemon Balm. Use any or all the herbs, place in the center of a square piece of cheesecloth or cotton, and tie up tight with string or wrap tightly with a rubber band. Throw the sachet into the bath under hot running water.

Melatonin

Hundreds of studies have shown a link between low Melatonin levels and cancer. Back in 1988, the results of a study published in the American Association for Cancer Research reported Melatonin slowed breast cancer cell proliferation between sixty to seventy-eight percent (Hill & Blask, 1988).

At the 2003 annual meeting of the American Association for Cancer Research, scientist David E. Blask reported, "the nighttime hormone melatonin puts breast cancer cells to sleep. It also slows breast cancer growth by seventy percent . . . when mice were subjected to constant light their tumor growth skyrocketed" (DeNoon, 2003).

Reported in 2010 in *ScienceDirect.com*, a nine year study with many groups and strains of aged male mice, dietary melatonin significantly reduced the size and number of tumors (Sharman, 2010).

Melatonin, a potent antioxidant, slowly drips out of your tiny pineal gland, inside your brain, as soon as darkness begins to fall. Melatonin is also produced in the retinas of your eyes, your skin, gastrointestinal tract and other organs.

This hormone regulates your body's sleep wake cycle. When light reaches your eyes in the morning, your pineal gland's Melatonin production slows, and you begin to wake.

To help raise your natural levels of Melatonin, get lots of restful sleep during darkness. Turn off all lights, including those from clock radios, computers and other electronics and use a sleeping mask if needed.

Several foods carry small amounts of Melatonin naturally, including: onions, cherries, bananas, corn, oats, rice, mint, lemon verbena, sage, thyme, feverfew and red wine, and the highest levels were found in rice.

Head of the study, Professor Darío Acuña Castroviejo, from the Universidad de Granada, states, "However, while the substance becomes legalized (*in Granada*), humans should try to increase melatonin consumption through food" (University of Granada, 2007).

High levels of Melatonin were found in Feverfew, St. John's Wort and Huang-qin (Scutellaria baicalensis) (Hardeland & Poeggeler, 2003).

EAT YOUR MELATONIN!

Very Rich Sources
Huang-qin
St. John's Wort
Feverfew

Rich Sources
White & Black Mustard Seeds
Wolfberry Seed
Fenugreek Seed
Almond Seed
Sunflower Seed
Fennel Seed
Alfalfa Seed
Green Cardamom seed
Flax Seed
Tart Monmorency Cherries
Extra Virgin Olive Oil

Moderate Sources
Anise Seed
Coriander Seed
Celery Seed
Poppy Seed
Milk Thistle Seed
Oat Seed
Onions
Bananas
Radishes
Tomatoes
Ginger
Corn
Oats
Rice
Mint
Lemon verbena
Sage
Thyme
Red wine & Beer (Phewf!)

(Hardeland & Pandi-Perumal, 2005; Reiter & Tan, 2002; University of Granada, 2007; Marcello, Varoni, Vitalini, 2010).

This explains why eating fresh Feverfew leaves when a headache is coming on causes you to feel verrrrry sleepy . . . zzzzzzzz. With a bitter and very distinctive flavour, Feverfew is also a beautiful herb when in bloom, with hundreds of tiny white flowers. A pretty and most useful herb to grow in your garden.

Melatonin shows anti-angiogenic factors, as well as immunomodulating, anti-oxidant, cytodifferentiating and anti-proliferative effects (Lissoni, Rovelli, Malugani, Bucovec, Conti, & Maestroni, 2001).

Melatonin supplementation is recommended by Alternative Practitioners to help cancer patients sleep better and boost levels of the cancer fighting molecule.

Synthetic Melatonin is made from crushing the pituitary glands of cows, pigs or other animals. This is not a safe practice and could expose you to dangerous viruses. Please make sure your Melatonin supplements are always made from food. Tart Montmorency Cherry Concentrate, is one of the world's finest sources of Melatonin. The Montmorency cherry is also a rich source of antioxidants. Immunotec's cherry concentrate is 100% pure and natural with no preservatives, additives, color or sweeteners. See the Resources section at the back of this book.

Alternative Healing Modalities

Consider the services of a relaxing healing modality such as Reiki, Massage Therapy or Reflexology. Many services are covered by benefit programs, but if you are not part of a plan, most practitioners have reasonable fees.

Reiki and some of the simpler techniques of Reflexology can be performed on you by loved ones or even by yourself. Reiki is a simple, natural and safe therapy that anyone can learn. Reiki uses our unseen life force energy to create a beneficial healing effect. Reiki Practitioners use this Japanese healing modality, known as 'laying on of hands' to reduce stress and relax your body.

Reflexology manipulates the zones in your hands and feet to relieve any stress you may be carrying, improve the circulation of your blood and lymph fluids and promote your overall health and wellbeing.

Reflexologists use their thumbs and fingers to walk over and between the bones and joints of your hands and feet. It is extremely relaxing and when performed properly, never hurts. Practitioners use methods such as walking, rotating, pressing, holding and tapping on your feet and hands, to trigger healing in corresponding areas of your body. For instance, healing of your colon can be triggered by pressure points down the bottom, outside of your feet; or your sciatic nerve responds to touch on the bottom of your heels (Voner, 2003).

Massage Therapy is performed by Registered Massage Therapists, who are well trained in all aspects of anatomy and function. Jennifer McGill, Registered Massage Therapist and Massage Therapy Instructor states:

Massage Therapy improves all body systems because it improves blood flow, which helps promote proper functioning of the body. If your muscles are too tight and pull on your spinal cord, they pull the vertebrae that line up to make the canal for your spinal cord. This pressure on your spinal cord, affects function of your central and peripheral nervous systems. When you have nerve compression, you don't have proper function.

Muscles can become so tense they compress blood vessels where they pass through. Massage therapy helps to work out this compression and tenseness, and improves circulation in both lymph and blood flow, improving all systems of your body.

Jennifer McGill, RMT, Massage Therapy Instructor, 2010.

Yoga Asanas

Asanas are one of the eight practices of Yoga. The other practices are: The Five Restraints – non-harming, truthfulness, non-stealing, moderation of the senses, and non-possessiveness; The Five Observances – purity, contentment, self-discipline, self-study, and self-surrender; Control and Expansion of Energy, Sense Withdrawal, Concentration, Meditation and Self-Realization (Anderson & Sovik, 2000).

Asanas are the poses we have come to know as Yoga. Practicing Asanas helps to clear your mind, detoxify your tissues and keep your body limber and young. It makes you slow down, discard the stresses of the day and go within to nurture your soul and create calm.

The Sun Salutation or Surya Namaskara is a series of twelve classic postures performed in a single, graceful flow. This Asana sequence builds strength and increases flexibility. You can do it anytime you need energy

202

or creative inspiration! Perform the Sun Salutation in a flowing movement, inhaling as you stretch and exhaling as you contract. You may do the sequence as many times as you wish. There are many, many versions of the Sun Salutation!

Simple Sun Salutation

Mountain Pose ~ Stand with your feet hip width apart, your hands by your sides or folded together at your chest, in prayer position.

Overhead Stretch ~ Inhale and sweep your arms up overhead, with palms facing, reaching, stretching tall, lift your chest, look up, keeping the back of your neck long.

Forward Bend ~ Exhale and with belly lock on, lengthen your spine, fold forward and grasp your ankles, or touch the floor, keeping knees bent or straight if you want more, touching your head to your knees.

Lunge Pose with Left Foot Forward ~ Step back with your right foot, placing knee on the floor if needed, placing your hands on either side of your front foot. Breathe into the pose, allowing your pelvis to sink to the floor on the out-breath.

Plank Pose ~ Stretch your left foot back, in line with your right, knees on the floor, turn your toes under and lift your knees into Plank Pose. Stay strong and straight from head to toe, like a plank, arms strong, hands facing forward. Hold as long as is comfortable.

Eight Limbs Pose ~ Lower your knees, your chest, then your forehead, keep your hips up, arms close to your sides.

Cobra Pose ~ Inhale, lowering your body to the floor, press your pelvis down into the floor, lift up and back, drawing your shoulders back and together, keeping hands flat on the floor, fingers pointing forward, arms close to your sides, looking forward.

Downward Dog Pose ~ On an exhale, press hands into the floor, turn toes under and lift your pelvis up and back, keeping your legs straight and pressing down with your heels, flattening and straightening your back.

Lunge Pose with Right Foot Forward ~ Inhale and step your right foot forward and place it between your hands, align your knee over your ankle, and extend your left leg behind, breathe into the stretch.

Forward Bend ~ Step forward with your left foot, with belly lock on, lift your pelvis, straighten your legs, lengthen your spine, folding forward, grasping your ankles, or touching the floor, keeping knees bent or straight if you want more.

Overhead Stretch ~ On an inhalation, bend your knees, sweep your arms up the sides and overhead, lengthening your spine, palms facing each other, stretching to the sky.

Mountain Pose ~ Exhale into mountain pose, hands in prayer, relaxed, calm, stay here quietly as long as you wish (Anderson & Sovik, 2000).

Wellness Spas

Therapeutic treatments at a spa can help relax and rejuvenate you. Combine with a nurturing setting in nature, and you have a place to cleanse and protect your physical body, nourish your soul and emotional body and strengthen your connection to self, spirit and the universe.

A Wellness Spa can offer cleansing seaweed wraps, nourishing vegetarian or vegan fare, relaxing spa treatments and a chance to reconnect and spend time with nature.

Where on earth would you find such a place? Nurturing wellness spas are all over the world, and you will find one in your area if you look hard enough. Near Toronto, Canada, about two hours north, you will find an incredible lakeside sanctuary for total healing, Grail Springs Body Mind Spirit Retreat and Spa.

If you cannot get to Grail Springs in the near future, you may want to read Madeleine Marentette's, *Grail Spring's Holistic Detox*. Owner, Madeleine Marentette shares her story of healing and the birth of Grail Springs. See the Resources section at the back of this book.

This is an excellent book on detoxing with detailed information about acid/alkaline balance, three and seven day detox diets, cleansing mineral baths and over seventy recipes from the Grail Springs kitchen.

On to the last principle, which engages common sense and greatly reduces the risk of overloading your body with toxins and creating disease . . .

Deep breathing alkalizes the body, while short breathing acidifies the body.

Madeleine Marentette, *Grail Spring's Holistic Detox*, 2007.

45 Principle 10 ~ Avoid The Causes ~ No, Everything Does Not Cause Cancer!

What does cause cancer anyway?

In 1775, Percival Pott, an eighteenth century London physician, described scrotal cancers in chimney sweeps. The soot left on their clothing and skin soon caused tumors on their scrotum (Waldron, 1983).

During the nineteenth century, history recorded many incidences of cancers caused by radiation and chemicals, including lung cancer in German miners; skin tumors and leukemias in people working with and patients receiving x-rays; tongue cancer in women who painted luminescent hands on wristwatches (from licking the paintbrush into a point), and by the 1950s, lung cancers in smokers started appearing in substantial numbers (Weinberg, 1998).

By the 1960s, scientists developed the ability to induce cancer in lab animals. Hundreds of chemicals were registered as causing mutagenic changes in the cells of lab animals (Weinberg, 1998).

Unfortunately this information was not related to humans because although we can induce cancer in, then *sacrifice* a test animal, such studies are not allowed to be performed on humans. But . . . isn't that exactly what we are doing by allowing cancer causing chemicals and radiation to be all around us, in our environment, in our homes and in our bodies? We are living in a giant cancer experiment!

Perhaps now, if we acknowledge the cancer causing effects of chemicals and radiation, we can hope the short, tortured lives of laboratory animals at least accounts for something. Hopefully, we can acknowledge that our lack of action to eliminate the cancer causing substances in our everyday life has had a devastating impact on our lives and our world, and finally do something about it.

We know that solvents, chemicals, synthetic hormones, chemotherapy, tobacco smoke, pesticides and radiation cause cancer and it just makes sense to eliminate cancer-causing substances from use.

When Lindane, a dangerous carcinogenic organochlorine and two other cancer-causing pesticides were banned from use in Israel, breast cancer rates immediately dropped between eight and thirty-four percent, after they had been rising steadily for twenty-five years! (Spangler, 1996).

In other countries, including all over North America, Lindane is used every day by mothers and children! Lindane is the pesticide found in the widely used pediculosis or lice shampoo.

Although Lindane has been banned in 52 countries and received an international ban in agricultural use from the Stockholm Convention on Persistent Organic Pollutants, *and* is known to be a carcinogen, it is still allowed to be used on the heads of North American children!

This product has been banned in the U.K. for some time now, but is still widely used in Canada and the United States (Stockholm Convention on Persistent Organic Pollutants, 2007).

The focus for cancer research clearly needs to be on prevention. Remove the causes and we will not have to deal with the fallout. When mutagenic compounds are no longer forced on us and nutrition is put back into our food, most cancer cases will never happen.

It is time for governments to take responsibility for the carcinogenic chemicals they allow to be used and manufacturers to take responsibility for the utmost safety of their products. As consumers it is time to become informed about the products we use and refuse to buy anything that contains chemicals and synthetics.

The information about the carcinogenicity of the chemicals we use is readily available. The International Agency for Research on Cancer (IARC) is part of the World Health Organization. Their mission is to "coordinate and conduct research on the causes of human cancer, the mechanisms of carcinogenesis, and to develop scientific strategies for cancer control." You can research any suspect chemical on the IARC website, and so can the manufacturers who make the products we use and the politicians who make the laws about the chemicals we use (IARC, 2010). Here: http://www.iarc.fr/

If we stop buying foods and products produced and packaged with dangerous chemicals, manufacturers will be forced to change their processes and produce safer products without the chemicals and additives which we refuse to buy!

Personal Care Products
Label reading is a necessary safety precaution when buying personal care products. This is one area where we are exposed to carcinogens on a regular basis. Manufacturers can put just about anything they want in their products. There are really no laws to protect consumers from dangerous and carcinogenic ingredients.

A study produced by the Environmental Working Group found hormone altering chemicals in teen makeup products. Hormones are a regular additive to personal care products like make-up, shampoo, conditioner and lotions. Livestock and in some cases human placentas are used by cosmetics manufacturers, who add them to products to impart skin softening qualities. Unfortunately, the manufacturers don't care that placentas have high levels of hormones which can cause reproductive problems for consumers! These products cause endocrine disruption and organ system toxicity (Sutton, 2008).

In the fall of 2005, Canada passed a law requiring all personal care products to be fully labeled on the outer container. When a similar law was passed in the United Kingdom it gave consumers the power to choose safe products over unsafe ones. It forced manufacturers to produce products without dangerous chemicals because now consumers could tell the difference, and the chemical laden products were being left on shelves.

Some manufacturers continue to try fooling consumers by printing the labels so small that it is impossible to read them without a magnifying glass. When I come across a product with very small printing, I immediately put the product back on the shelf. It makes me think the manufacturer has something to hide.

Skin Deep is a project of the Environmental Working Group. The *Skin Deep Cosmetic Safety Database* is an excellent resource for most personal care products. I checked my daughter Anna's de-frizzing product. Every morning I listen to her humming away innocently while running Sunsilk de frizz through her gorgeous long curly hair. Here's what I found:

The manufacturer of Sunsilk de frizz, Unilever, has not signed The Environmental Working Group's, Campaign for Safe Cosmetics, a voluntary pledge to formulate products that don't use ingredients that are suspected or known to cause certain health concerns.

This manufacturer, Unilever, conducts animal testing. Ingredients from packaging: Water - Aqua, Cyclopentasiloxane, Polyquaternium-37, Isopropyl Myistate, Cetearyl Alcohol, Polyquaternium-4, Propylene Glycol Dicaprylate/Dicaprate, Fragrance - Parfum, Behentrimonium Chloride, Glyceryl Stearate, DMDM Hydantoin, PPG-1 Trideceth-6, Propylene Glycol, Tocopheryl Acetate - Vitamin E Acetate, Tetrasodium EDTA, Iodopropynyl Butylcarbamate, Aloe Barbadensis Leaf Extract - Aloe Vera, Sorbitol, Algae Extract, Yellow 5 - CI 19140, Green 3 - CI 42053.

The ingredients in this product are linked to:
✓ Use restrictions
✓ Allergies/immunotoxicity
✓ Other concerns for ingredients used in this product:

Neurotoxicity, Persistence and bioaccumulation, Organ system toxicity
(Non-reproductive), Miscellaneous, Irritation (skin, eyes, or lungs),
Enhanced skin absorption, Contamination concerns, Occupational hazards.

Use the *Skin Deep Cosmetic Safety Database* to check the products in your cupboard. You will be amazed and disgusted at what you will find lurking in innocent, fresh and natural looking packages. Here: http:// www.ewg.org/skindeep/

Synthetic Hormones

Synthetic hormones in birth control pills and hormone replacement therapy also contribute to reproductive cancers. The *Women's Health Initiative* is a massive fifteen year study that definitively proved the link between synthetic hormones like those in hormone replacement therapy and birth control; and reproductive cancers, especially breast cancer. The study also proved risks for heart disease, stroke and blood clots (Women's Health Initiative, 2010). Here: www.nhlbi.nih.gov/whi/

Make your living environment a chemical-free zone as much as possible. Find safer alternatives for soaps, shampoos, fragrances, cleaners and disinfectants. Avoid furniture with excessive adhesives and plastics and stick with solid wood wherever possible.

Avoid nylon, plastic and other synthetic fabrics and choose natural fabrics instead. Never use pesticides, fungicides or herbicides in or around your home. Remove extra cans of solvents, paints and stains to reduce off gassing. Throw out all plastic food containers and use glass, stainless steel or other inert containers.

Healing takes time and awareness. Just follow the 10 healing principles. Begin by adding nurturing foods and lifestyle changes, letting them gradually become an integral part of your life, while you move past damaging foods, products and behaviors.

In this way you will *not* feel deprived; instead you will feel powerful, rejuvenated and on the path of healing . . .

In the 1990s Chandra Tiwary, a retired endocrinologist from the Brooks Military Base in Texas, kept seeing black babies with breasts. Girls as young as one and as old as three were showing up with breast growth and pubic hair . . . all the mothers had regularly applied creams to their babies' heads to smooth their hair. These creams contained various ingredients touted for the ability to get rid of frizz. Sometimes they were labeled as containing placenta, estriol or hormones. When the parents stopped using the creams, their babies' breasts went away.

Devra Davis, *The Secret History Of The War On Cancer,* 2007.

46 Escharotics

Enter . . . Greg Caton and Cansema®.

Backing up a bit, in 2008, I made several enquiries into whether people would be interested in being interviewed for a documentary film on the truth about cancer. I came across Cansema® Black Salve on HerbHealers.com, emailed the owner Greg Caton and asked if he would be interested in my project. He sent me an email saying he was very interested, and I could interview him at his home outside of the United States, where he was living with his wife and child. He didn't reveal where he lived. At that time, I was not ready to do the interview, but was considering the level of interest in such a project.

I had *truth shivers*, as I read his email, realizing that he was living outside of the U.S. for legal reasons, associated with the manufacture and distribution of herbal products that cure cancer. A little research on the internet showed Greg was incarcerated in the United States for selling *drugs*. He went to jail for thirty-three months, then moved to Ecuador on his release.

The truth, I felt, was *not* that Greg Caton is a criminal, but that Greg Caton is a *genius*. Thousands of people have purchased and been healed by Cansema® Black Salve and his other products. You can read and see hundreds of testimonials on his website and throughout the internet.

In early 2010, I receive an email from Mike Adams and Natural News linking to an article, 'FDA dupes Interpol to achieve illegal kidnapping and deportation of herbal formulator Greg Caton.' Greg Caton has been arrested in Ecuador. At gunpoint, in a staged road block, he is handcuffed and taken to a holding facility to await a hearing. Conveniently, a few days before the scheduled hearing, he is forced on a plane to Miami by U.S. authorities. Before the plane has left, an Ecuadorian judge races to the airport and orders the U.S. pilot to release Greg Caton from the plane immediately, as they are violating Ecuadorian and international laws. The U.S. pilot ignores the judge and begins the flight to Miami (Adams, 2009).

At this time of writing, Greg Caton is awaiting trial in a Miami jail for continuing to sell what the FDA calls *drugs* . . . cancer curing herbal products that may have saved thousands of lives, Pattie MacDonald's included (more in a minute). In Ecuador, Greg Caton is allowed to say that his herbal preparation heals cancer and he is allowed to sell it. Ecuadorians embrace herbal medicine. Their constitution says that all citizens have access to natural medicines. They are allowed to use natural therapies that save their lives.

They are not forced to undergo life threatening, poisonous chemotherapy injections like Billy Best or the Canadian boy from Hamilton.

Mike Adam's detailed report can be found at, 'FDA dupes Interpol to achieve illegal kidnapping and deportation of herbal formulator Greg Caton' (Adams, 2009). Here: http://www.naturalnews.com/027750_Greg_Caton_FDA.html

Mike Adams interviews Cathryn Caton (Greg's wife) and provides a free download of the mp3 on his website at, "Health Ranger Report #84: Greg Caton kidnapped, deported by FDA." Look down the list to find the audio report in mp3 format (Naturalnews.com, 2010). Here: http://www.naturalnews.com/Index-Podcasts.html

Greg Caton hasn't left us high and dry though. He writes Meditopia, his version of politics surrounding the *cancer sickness* industry. He distributes *Meditopia* freely, and asks that others download the entire book and attach it to their websites, so the information is never lost (Caton, 2006). Here: http://www.meditopia.org/

Then Greg produces a video that shows exactly how to make an escharotic preparation.

Escharotics are herbal medicines that cause an eschar, or scab to form, just as in Pattie's breast and neck tumor photos, coming up next. Escharotic salves cause the tumor to fester, then your immune system moves in and pushes the festering tumor out of healthy tissues below.

Escharotics have been suppressed, along with other cancer cures, for over one-hundred years, and Greg finds proof of many patents for escharotic formulations that were granted, then later suppressed (Caton, 2006).

Why would U.S. health authorities want to suppress the effectiveness of escharotics?

At this point, I'm sure you already know the answer, but if you don't, please . . .   read *Meditopia*. Here: www.meditopia.org/

It is late at night, I have been mesmerized by Greg Caton's videos on YouTube for hours. He shows exactly how to make an escharotic preparation with zinc butter or zinc chloride, and the herb Bloodroot. He gives another example with ninety percent Chaparral and ten percent other mixed herbs, which he does not disclose.

Only problem . . . you cannot get zinc chloride in Canada. It is considered a hazardous product and is tightly controlled. I call a Canadian supplier for zinc chloride and the receptionist tells me, "We can't just sell it to anybody . . . to work with in their kitchen or backyard!"

211

The Material Safety Data Sheet for Zinc Chloride or Zinc Butter states that it is extremely corrosive, causing burns to any area of contact. I can see why Greg Caton uses it to cause an infection at the site of a cancerous tumor. I can also see why he says of using the black salve, 'Use only as much as you need, a tiny amount. Follow the directions closely . . . more is not better.'

Chaparral is also known as Stinkweed, for its foul odour. Mexicans call it Hediondilla, which means '*little stinker.*' It has been used for many years by Native Americans for treatment of snake bites, sores, burns, chicken pox, arthritis, and bronchitis, and later by pioneers for the treatment of stomach, liver and kidney cancers. The active ingredient is NDGA or nordihydroguaiaretci acid, a powerful antioxidant which kills bacteria and other microorganisms (Reader's Digest, 1998).

Bloodroot also has a rich history of medicinal use by Native Americans and natural practitioners. In *The Way Of Herbs*, Michael Tierra reports, "Bloodroot is used in a black paste salve for removing tumors, skin cancers, moles and other topical excrescences" (Tierra, 1998).

Zinc Chloride in a paste along with herbs like Chaparral and Bloodroot, literally burns through your skin, causing your immune system to react, a boiling infection to ensue and anything that is *not you* is expelled.

Escharotic Preparations - Intro by Greg Caton, Part 1 of 3
Watch at http://www.youtube.com/watch?v=9XaZlYbxGek

Escharotic Preparations - Intro by Greg Caton, Part 2 of 3
Watch at http://www.youtube.com/watch?v=PmdstCSyDqs&NR=1

Escharotic Preparations - Intro by Greg Caton, Part 3 of 3
Watch at http://www.youtube.com/watch?v=qgmQV5UgeDw&NR=1

Without the ability to purchase Zinc Chloride, I wonder if it is needed anyway?

I know my formula causes a festering reaction, without the pain and eschar. It works slower, is much gentler and painfree. I have tested it on melanoma, basal cell carcinoma, cysts, weird changing dark moles and other strange growths – it got rid of everything, slowly but surely – and it works on internal cancers as well! I have been working away at a large cyst on the side of my leg.

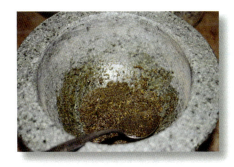

Bitter Tonic Herbs with olive oil

The cyst is almost two centimeters wide and close to one centimeter high. It popped up one day, literally. I never noticed it, and then all of a sudden there it was!

Curiously, it showed up after I started eating dairy products for a short period, and after a bit of research, I find a link between consumption of dairy and the appearance of cysts. The herbs are crushed and mixed with a small amount of olive oil. Sometimes I use fresh juice from my aloe plant. The paste is stored in a glass jar in the refrigerator. It is pasted on the cyst, taped it with a bandage, and left overnight.

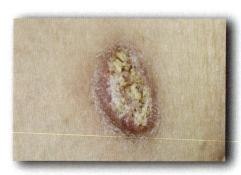

Like always, the herbal mixture causes festering as it eats away at the inside of the cyst, which incidentally is a white, foamy mass, somewhat like yeast . . . Can you see how the herbal mixture causes the top layer of the cyst to fester, then dry up and fall off?

After about fifteen applications the cyst is almost gone.

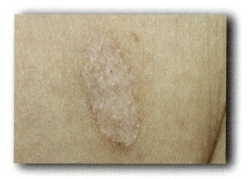

Now there is only a scar where the large cyst used to be.

47 Escharotics Cure Breast Cancer

The Cancer Journal ~ Heal Yourself! is almost finished but something is holding me back. I blame myself for dragging my feet. As always, with patience, the reason soon becomes evident.

I have been saving studies, reports, articles, testimonials and information for over ten years now; that is how I know so many others have healed themselves. I come across a brief testimonial from a woman named Pattie. She claims to have cured cancerous breast tumors with Cansema®. She bought the escharotic preparation through a friend. I contact her by email and at first she is hesitant to talk to me. When Pattie realizes I am not a threat to her, she generously offers her story of breast cancer, and photographs of the eschars produced by Cansema®, and the subsequent cure of all her breast and neck tumors.

Pattie tells me that in late 2002, her phone was tapped and she was contacted by Quackwatch.org under false pretenses, "In regard to my cancer . . . I don't know what their intentions were; but I had a gut feeling it was not good."

Where do I start? As I look back I realized my cancer was a long, hard journey; but the end results: happy, healthy and alive. I did not only cure my cancer; I had irritable bowel, sinus infection, carpel tunnel and a few other ills.

I am not a physician; however, I believe my body was slowly shutting down in 2002. At one point, before I met Greg Caton, I laid on my couch and wanted to die, I was so sick. Then, my grandmother called me from Illinois (she was 101 at that time). She told me to put all of my prescription drugs in the trash, change my diet and so on. Within a week of following her advice, I started to feel better; but I still had to deal with my breast cancer.

My cancer surgeon had scheduled me for breast surgery on a Tuesday in June and I had to confront the fact that I was possibly going to lose my entire breast (cried a lot). My right breast had a lump the size of a quarter according to the ultrasound and the biopsy was inconclusive for cancer. They wanted to cut on me and had no concrete tests.

Despite this emotional roller coaster my doctor had me on, I decided to trust her and go forward with the surgery – didn't think I had any other choice. I am naively allowing doctors to take control of my health.

Then, my new life begins: a friend of many years, who I hadn't spoken to in over a year, calls me on the Sunday before my surgery. She had heard from another friend about my upcoming breast surgery and asked to meet with me immediately and to cancel my surgery for the time being.

A few months back I had started a learning session on meditation and regressing into my past lives (what a wonderful trip). The reason I mention this: I know now it had everything to do with my cancer journey. I was being led to the right people at the right time to literally save my life.

At this point I am also extremely curious about how she healed herself of ovarian cancer without Western medical intervention. I meet with my friend at a motel – it was about half-way between our houses, because of the long distance. Also, she was taking care of her sister at the time, who was doing chemo and needed looking after. Sadly, her sister died in September after doing chemo, she was fifty-one. Her sister trusted her doctors and wanted nothing to do with natural medicine, changing her diet, etc.

Anyway, she shows me photos of her ovarian cancer tumors (dead and black) literally falling out of her and I am in awe. I know and trust this woman; so I decide to go for it.

Besides, what do I have to lose and I might just be able to save my breast. She proceeds to remove the biopsy scab, applied Cansema and bandages me up.

It has only been a few hours after applying the Cansema; but, my right breast is so painful, I cannot go back to sleep. Deb told me it was going to be painful; but this is worse than childbirth.

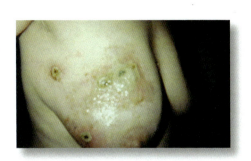

I have no choice but to take a pain pill and then realize I trashed all of my prescriptions. I took the only thing I had left--aspirin. Needless to say, I spent two days in bed, in pain with little sleep. I comforted myself in believing this was better than losing my breasts and it was. However, in the future, I will know to have pain meds on hand.

On the third day the sharp pains are subsiding and the pain is now a dull, aching pain--not so bad. Deb told me to take daily photos; which I did. She explained that nobody would believe I ever had cancer if I didn't have proof.

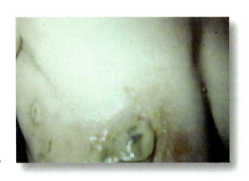

On the tenth day this thing, which was the size of a half dollar, was ready to fall off and I am freaking out.

216

*Decide I need a bath –
that may relax me. I
was freaking, because I
know nothing about
natural medicines/
herbs and thought I
might bleed to death
when the tumor falls*

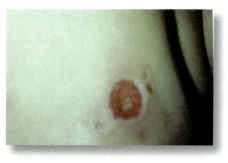

*off. Have my cordless phone on the floor in the bathroom;
just in case I need to call 911. Looking back, my fear was so
unwarranted.*

*The tumor fell off and I decided to save it--more proof. No
bleeding, no pain and I feel absolutely wonderful. During
this ten day period, I had two pimples on my neck and they
were itching terribly. Deb told me to apply Cansema on
them and wait and watch.*

*Sure enough I had
cancer somewhere in
my neck area.
Strange, because I
had been going to a
specialist for my neck
pains and sinus
infections for over a
year. What did he do?
Nothing, gave me pain*

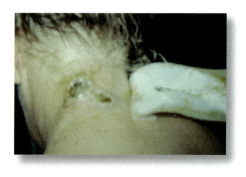

*pills and steriods. I had also been losing my ability to grasp
anything with my left hand and dropped stuff all the time.*

*The two pimples were on the left side of my neck. I applied
the Cansema and bandaged my neck. This pain was not
sharp; but dulling – not bad at all.*

The neck tumors, the size of a dime, fell off in about ten days. There are a few scars; but hardly noticeable. I went to Greg's website and decided to order the Cansema tonic and took it for a 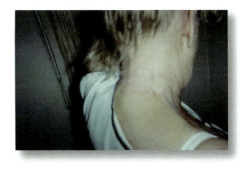 *few months on Greg's recommendation. I was also in contact with Jason Vale at this time. I needed supplement and diet recommendations. I cannot believe I am being led to people who I need to be alive and well.*

While my neck tumors were festering, still naive and wanting proof my breast cancer was gone, I make an appointment with my general doctor. She flips out when she takes my 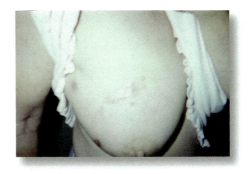 *neck bandages off and insists on calling my son for permission to put me in a cancer clinic. What is her problem--she thinks I am nuts, I am guessing. Really confused at this point. I refuse to give her my son's phone number and leave her office in tears.*

I did manage to get a few jars of formaldehyde from her to preserve my breast tumor. Told her I was going to bring it to her for tests; but decided to never go back to her, ever.

Long story shortened, I later went to the county hospital for mammogram, blood tests, etc. and didn't tell them anything when asked about my scars. All tests done – negative.

At this point, I am really confused and cannot understand why doctors are not using this for cancer. Thus, my research into natural medicine begins. The first book I read is "Politics in Healing" by Daniel Haley.

My awesome angels must be working overtime again . . .

„

Pattie MacDonald, 2010.

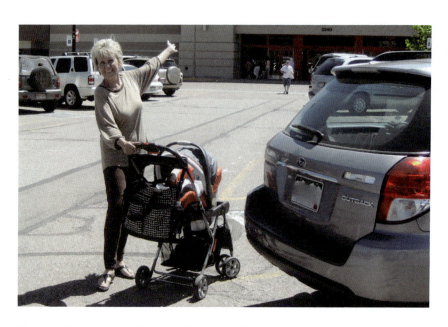

Pattie ~ Happy and Healthy in 2010, eight years after curing herself!

Heal Yourself! . . .

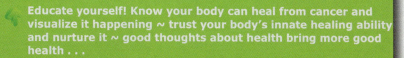

Educate yourself! Know your body can heal from cancer and visualize it happening ~ trust your body's innate healing ability and nurture it ~ good thoughts about health bring more good health . . .

Be in tune with your body and listen to your own messages ~ which come to you as symptoms . . .

Cleanse your blood, tissues and organs ~ detoxify your body of damaged fats, pathogens, debris, acids, cholesterol build up, chemicals and harmful toxins ~ Download Cleanse Your Body!, to start healing now ~ Go to **www.thegoodwitch.ca/start-with-cleanses-first/** . . .

Eat anti fungal foods like raw onions, ginger, garlic or garlic pills, and dried or raw aromatic culinary herbs like oregano, sage and thyme added to food just before serving . . .

Use anti-cancer herbal teas like turmeric, red clover flower, burdock leaf or root, dandelion root, green tea and anti-cancer herbal medicines like Bitter Tonic Tea™, Harry Hoxsey's tea, Essiac™ or your own similar blend, internally or externally as needed . . .

Eat fresh, raw, organic fruits and vegetables and green smoothies that make you feel amazing and alive ~ sea vegetables like nori, kombu and kelp, Swiss chard and other greens, undenatured proteins from raw foods, natural supplementation, more raw food . . .

Eat fresh, raw, organic nuts and seeds and their highly unsaturated oils, especially flax and hemp, rich in cancer fighting Omega 3, up to 3 tablespoons of oil daily ~ add olive oil to food after it is cooked ~ make your own salad dressings with fresh cold pressed organic oils ~ get started with simple, delicious recipes at Salad Strategies ~ Go to **www.thegoodwitch.ca/salad-strategies/** . . .

Eat organic whole grains, raw and soaked or cooked al dente, including organic steel cut or large oats with focus on non gluten grains such as brown rice, quinoa, amaranth and millet, fresh raw sprouts, lentils, peas and beans . . .

Breathe deeply, yoga, tai chi, walk, move, grow your own food, meditate, be with nature, get a suntan, laugh, learn, research, read, take time for yourself, rest, be still, be grateful, enjoy music, holidays, playing, eating, family, loving, living . . .

Learn how others have healed, hear, read and see their stories, then mirror what works for you ~ go to **www.IncredibleHealingJournals.com**

49   Initiate & Promote Cancer...

Believing old paradigms ~ that your body cannot heal ~ that chemotherapy, radiation and surgery are the only way ~ that toxic drugs, radiation exposure and synthetic supplements are better for you than fresh, nutritious, organic food and herbs, air, water, sunshine, movement and love . . .

Giving up your power ~ believing that you have no control over your body and its healing capabilities . . .

Stress, worry, fear, anxiety, buying into fear mongering, negative thoughts, thoughts about illness attract more illness . . .

Mmmmm, cancer cells love sugar in all forms, high fructose corn syrup, glucose, sucrose, pastries, French fries, baked goods, bread, cake, donuts, croissants, soda pop, beer, wine, spirits, and refined white pasta, corn, rice and wheat . . .

Acid causing high protein animal foods, cooked foods, pasteurized dairy products, animal flesh and excess refined grains ~ makes for an acidic, sweet, oxygen-less environment ~ perfect for fungi . . .

Synthetic hormones like those in birth control pills, hormone replacement therapies, estrogen like chemicals from plastics coming in contact with food or water, commercially grown livestock fed growth hormones to increase milk or meat production, beef, pork, turkey, chicken . . .

Nutritional deficiencies . . .

Hydrogenated and damaged trans-configured fats found in shortening, partially hydrogenated fat, and cooked vegetable oils in all fried foods, crackers, cookies, fast foods, frozen foods and baked goods, charred foods . . .

Packaged, fried, frozen and fast foods and foods with chemicals like aspartame, saccharin, preservatives, artificial dyes and flavors, chlorinated and fluoridated water . . .

Chemicals in personal care products, dry cleaning, household and industrial cleaning products ~ plastics, solvents, Teflon coatings, heavy metals like mercury, lead and cadmium . . .

Radiation exposure including medical radiation in mammograms, CT scans, bone scans, thyroid scans, dental xrays, barium enemas, too much sun exposure without adequate nutrition, chemotherapy, toxic chemicals, pesticides, herbicides, fungicides, smoking, chronic acid indigestion from congested liver and gallbladder, removal of gallbladder, acid blood, black mold and other fungi like aflatoxins in peanuts and grains, and Candida Albicans . . .

50 The Value Of Suffering

We shall draw from the heart of suffering itself the means of inspiration and survival.

Winston Churchill.

I think Winston Churchill knew the value of suffering.

Have you ever thought about the value of suffering? I mean, how much is it worth? In money? No amount could possibly be worth the unnecessary suffering of another human being. What about a child? How much would the suffering of a child be worth?

I wonder about suffering. I think about what my mother gave up so we could learn NOT to do what she did. I think about what a gift it was that my father unknowingly handed over his spleen and kidney and suffered terribly for over nine years so that others could learn NOT to do what he did.

We all know and understand the deception around cancer. Don't you think it is time we stopped lying to ourselves and lived our truths instead?

Then we can all stop suffering . . .

Remember the Oncology nurse?

With tears in her eyes, in front of someone she had never met, Fran acknowledged the truth, of how she feels about the *treatment* administered to sick cancer patients every day.

If the Nursing College heard what Fran had to say about her job, chances are she would be quickly dismissed from hospital employment and risk losing her nursing license.

I work nights so I don't have to hang chemotherapy bags . . . I hate it. I hate giving that shit to people. It's red poison going right into their bloodstream, right up into their brains . . . I'm so sick of the medical industry. It's all about money . . . all of it.

April 2010, Fran B., Registered Nurse, Oncology, Canada. Her name has been changed to protect her identity.

Fran spoke *her truth,* directly from her heart that day, her suffering fueled by the unnecessary loss of her mother, at the very hands of the system that pays her bills and puts food on her table.

Thank you Fran. We understand your inner turmoil and are grateful for your gift of truth.

51　The Cancer Revelations ~ Thank You Neale Donald Walsch!
(Author of the *Conversations With God* series)

The Old Revelations About Cancer

Present beliefs about cancer include a nightmare of toxic treatments and complete denial of the pivotal role of the patient in their own healing . . .

We believe cancer is a scourge on humanity, a deadly creeping crablike disease, eating away at our bodies, devastating our families and our lives . . .

We believe cancer arises from our own tissues, a body gone wrong . . .

We believe a large part of cancer is genetic – my mother had it why shouldn't I? My mother was always urging me to get a colonoscopy to make sure I didn't have colon cancer like her. In a defeated voice, one of the last things she said to me was, "Well, if I've got it, you'll probably get it too."

We believe cancer is a devastating disease, causing pain, discomfort, debilitation, sorrow, suffering and loss . . .

We believe doctors are the only people who know anything about cancer . . .

We believe if we start asking questions our doctor may disown us and we will be left to fend for ourselves . . .

We believe we have no role in healing our own cancer other than to sit in doctors' offices, waiting to be told what to do . . .

We believe chemotherapy, surgery and radiation are the only *proven* treatments available . . .

We believe our hair will fall out . . . our nails will fall off . . . we will vomit and become emaciated . . .

We believe we will suffer and die . . .

What are these beliefs based on?
They are based on fear and manipulation.

They are based on coercion and greed.

They are based on something someone else has told us.

Some others have a different story, as you have learned in this book.

What will be your story?
The story of devastation, pain and suffering?

Or . . . the story of the joy of life, healing and truth?

The New Revelations About Cancer

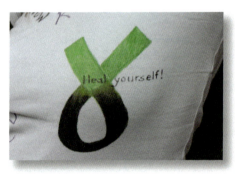

We are holding false beliefs about cancer that are not serving us, beliefs that are harming and killing us . . .

There are *healing truths* about cancer which have been revealed many times throughout history; they have all been denied, ridiculed and suppressed by greed . . .

Others have realized these *healing truths* and used the information to heal themselves . . .

Embracing these *healing truths* about cancer will help us immensely and reduce tremendous suffering for millions of people on our planet . . .

We *can* let go of old crippling beliefs and embrace these *new healing truths* about cancer . . .

We *can* make informed choices for ourselves and take responsibility for our actions, our health and our life . . .

We *can* help each other . . .

We *can* educate ourselves . . .

We *can* heal ourselves!

THANK YOU!

Thank You for buying this book and trusting me to offer valuable information.

I sincerely hope you use the information in this book to help your body heal.

I would be thrilled to hear how you have used the concepts and recipes in this or any of my books. You are welcome to send any comments to support@thegoodwitch.ca or use the contact form at www.thegoodwitch.ca/contact.

Please visit my website at www.thegoodwitch.ca where you will find more tools and tips for healing yourself.

Also, you may wish to visit www.incrediblehealingjournals.com to see remarkable stories of exactly how others have used key principles of healing to cure themselves.

Until next time,

Happy Healing!

Lisa

THE FAVOUR OF A REVIEW...

Reviews, ratings and comments on Amazon about this book are whole-heartedly appreciated. If you have enjoyed this visit into the world of making your own cancer medicines, you can leave a review by visiting this book's Amazon page when you're at a computer.

You'll also have a chance to rate the book and share your rating with your friends on Facebook and Twitter, after you turn the last page.

I read every review of my books and love to hear what readers have to say. It guides me to write books that are more likely to help others. If you have a moment, I'd be grateful for your time.

To find this book's page, search The Cancer Journal Heal Yourself on Amazon.com. Scroll down to Customer Reviews, and you will see a link on the right to 'Create Your Own Review'.

Thank You, Thank You, Thank You!

Appendix A: Medicinal Plants ~ Their Properties and Actions

Adaptogen ~ Adapt the body stress and reduce its effects

Alterative ~ Our welcome friends, alteratives are plants that deeply and gently cleanse our blood, while removing toxins and excess moisture. They stimulate our immune system to produce white blood cells and have been used in cancer therapies forever. They are best used consistently for a period of weeks or months. People debilitated by illness should start alteratives slowly, and gently increase the dose over a one to two week period. Their detoxifying action can cause systemic toxicity if the amount of waste and acids released from tissues is too much for the overburdened, eliminatory organs; the liver, skin, lungs, bowels and kidneys. North American natives used an astringent and healing alterative from the bark and twigs of the Alder tree. Made into a tea, herbs with the alterative quality, gently aid the body back to health by their action of general detoxification (Reader's Digest, 1998).

Analgesic ~ Pain relieving

Anthelmintic ~ Destroys parasitic worms

Anti-angiogenic ~ Reduces formation of new blood vessels. Used in cancer treatment with fewer side effects than chemotherapy.

Antibacterial ~ Destroys bacteria and inhibits their growth

Antibiotic ~ In natural or synthetic form, antibiotics are inherently designed to destroy microorganisms, or inhibit their growth, possess antibacterial properties.

Anti-Cancer ~ Works against cancer

Anticoagulant ~ Prevents or delays blood coagulation

Anti-diabetic ~ Prevents or relieves diabetes

Anti-diarrheal ~ Prevents diarrhea

Anti-fungal ~ Inhibits the growth of and destroys fungi

Anti-inflammatory ~ Counteracts inflammation

Anti-leukemic ~ Working against leukemia

Anti-mutagenic ~ Works against genetic mutations

Anti-nausea ~ Counteracts nausea

Antipyretic ~ Lowers fever

Anti-rheumatic ~ Works against rheumatism – acute and chronic condition of inflammation, muscle soreness, joint and bone pain.

Antispasmodic ~ Preventing or relieving spasm

Anti-tumor ~ Inhibits the growth of and destroys tumors

Anti-ulcer ~ Works against ulcers

Astringent ~ Constricting or binding effect

Bitter tonic ~ Bitter tasting medicine that increases strength and tone, stimulates appetite, improves digestion, and works to detoxify, cleanse and nourish tissues and fluids.

Calming ~ Works to calm and relax the nervous system and body, sedative, soothing.

Cancer preventive ~ Prevents the growth of cancer

Candidacide ~ Destroys Candida Albicans

Carminative ~ Prevents and relieves formation of gas in intestinal tract

Cathartic ~ Produces bowel movements

Demulcent ~ Demulcent herbs are easy to recognize by crushing the herb between your wet fingers. Demulcents become slippery like mucous, you can imagine how this slippery substance soothes irritated and inflamed tissues. They are used in herbal mixtures to soften and counteract the harsh properties of bitter herbs. While Cascara Sagrada will cause irritation through its generally harsh cathartic action, Licorice and Slippery Elm bark work to protect, soothe and heal, bringing balance to the formula and it's medicinal actions.

Deobstruent ~ Clears obstructions or blockages

Depurative ~ While the action of alteratives is on the body as a whole by draining and cleansing, the depurative plants work more specifically with the lymph, skin and blood to purify by eliminating waste and organic toxins. Barberry possesses depurative properties, assisting by purifying blood and lymph fluids (Vogel, 1970).

Diaphoretic ~ Increases perspiration

Digestive ~ Aids digestion

Diuretic ~ Increases urine secretion

Emetic ~ Induces vomiting

Emmenagogue ~ Promotes menstruation

Emollient ~ Softens and smoothes

Expectorant ~ Promotes clearance of mucous from respiratory tract

Fungicidal ~ Kills fungi and fungal spores

Hemostatic ~ Stops bleeding

Hepato protective ~ Protects the liver

Hypotensive ~ Lowers blood pressure

Immunostimulant ~ Stimulates the immune system

Laxative ~ Loosens the bowels

Lithotriptic ~ Dissolves stones

Mucolytic ~ Reduces thickness of sputum or mucous, liquifies

Nematicidal ~ Kills nematodes

Nervine ~ Calms the nervous system

Nutritive ~ A nourishing food source

Pro-estrogenic ~ A precursor of estrogen, metabolized into estrogen

Prophylactic ~ Contributes to the prevention of infection and disease

Purgative ~ Produces bowel movements

Rubefacient ~ Increases blood flow to the skin, causing redness

Sedative ~ Soothing, tranquilizing

Soothing lubricant ~ Reduces friction

Stimulant ~ Increases functional activity

Vulnerary ~ An herb used to heal wounds

Appendix B: Essential Recipes

For delicious healing
recipes go to
www.thegoodwitch.ca/
nutrition/

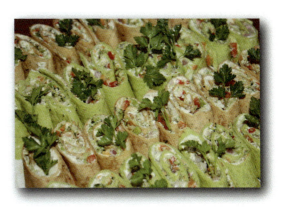

Healing foods taste
amazing! Here's a sample
of some of our delicious
healthy recipes at
TheGoodWitch.ca:

Antioxidant Rich Fragrant Chai Tea Blend ~ Make it yourself easy peasy
Asian Noodles ~ You won't be able to stop eating these noodles
Chai Green Smoothie ~ So creamy and Chai-y, mmmmm
Chocolate Strawberry Hemp Smoothie ~ Nothing goes better together
Cranberry Cleanser ~ You'll never buy Cranberry juice again
Easy Fresh Guacamole ~ Simple and quick and delicious
Heavenly Garlicky Hummus ~ You'll never buy hummus again
Hemp Milk and other easy Seed and Nut Milks ~ Healing milks
House Salad with Creamy Lime Dressing ~ Delish
Maple Spiced Candied Raw Nuts ~ So yummy and healing
Miso Soup ~ Traditional healing food
Orange Banana Smoothie ~ Tastes like a creamsicle
Party Veggie Roll Ups ~ Photo above ~ Great party food
Potassium Broth ~ Healing and nourishing therapeutic food
Raw Chocolate Cranberry Fudge ~ Rich and chocolatey
Raw Nori Handroll ~ Use your favourite veggies
Salad Strategies ~ Lots of ideas including Basic Vinaigrette, Basic
Balsamic, Sweet Honey Dijon Vinaigrette, Vivacious Vinaigrette,
Fabulous French and Gorgeous Greek Salad Dressing and Pasta Salad
Seasoned Multigrain Croutons ~ You'll never buy croutons again!
Soaking Beans and Peas ~ Simple and quick advice
Strawberry Fruit Leather ~ Kids absolutely love this
Sweet Potato Wedges and Chipotle Mayonnaise ~ One of our favourites

Appendix C: Essential Resources

Titles are links in the electronic version of this book. You may visit any resource by clicking on the title of each entry or on the full url in light blue below each description.

If you are reading the printed version of this book, you may visit any resource here by copying the full url address into your web browser on your computer or mobile device.

Adam's Website
Learn visualization techniques from a Molecular Biologist ~ Adam is a master of healing visualizations and teaches others through his incredible best selling books and sold out workshops.
www.dreamhealer.com/

Adam's Global Intention Heals Project
An experiment on the scientific proof on the effectiveness of visualization in healing. The project records the EEG brainwave measurements of a healee, to show the connection to that individual, while people at an Intention Heals workshop focus on healing a specific problem for her.
www.intentionheals.com/

Adam's Visualization DVD
Illustrates *exactly* how to use visualization techniques to heal your body and improve your life.
www.thegoodwitch.ca/bookshelf/

American Indian Medicine
Indian theories of disease, methods of treatment, early observations and the influence of indian medicine on folk medicine.
www.thegoodwitch.ca/bookshelf/

Anti-angiogenesis ~ Eat To Defeat Cancer
www.eattodefeat.org/evidence

Anti-angiogenesis ~ William Li: Can we eat to starve cancer? ~ Video
Dr. William Li speaks on Ted, Ideas Word Spreading, Dr. William Li discusses Angiogenesis and foods that have anti-angiogenetic properties, that cut off the blood supply to tumors.
www.thegoodwitch.ca/can-we-eat-to-starve-cancer-video/

Ani Phyo ~ Ani's Raw Food Kitchen

One of the best raw chefs on the planet . . . amazing cookbooks.
www.thegoodwitch.ca/bookshelf/

Ani Phyo ~ Ani's Raw Food Desserts: 85 Delectable Sweets and Treats

One of the best raw chefs on the planet – Amazing cookbooks!
www.thegoodwitch.ca/bookshelf/

Apoptosis and Signal Transduction

An amazing animation of the process of Apoptosis, where a cell self destroys after interaction with a Natural Killer Cell.
www.wehi.edu.au/education/wehitv/apoptosis_and_signal_transduction/

Arm & Hammer ~ Antacid

Will Baking Soda Work As An Antacid?
www.armhammer.com/basics/magic/

Back to Eden

Jethro Kloss wrote Back To Eden way back in the early 1970s. It is full of simple and timeless remedies.
www.thegoodwitch.ca/bookshelf/

Billy Best Interview

Mike Adams interviews Billy Best on fleeing from Chemotherapy treatments at age 16 to beat Hodgkins Lymphoma naturally.
www.NaturalNews.com/026337_cancer_Billy_Best_chemotherapy.html

Billy Best's Website

Learn more about Billy's story, or support Billy by purchasing Essiac™ through his website.
www.billybest.net/index.htm

Billy Best Speaks About Danny Hauser, Part 1

Mike Cann.net interviews Billy Best about Danny Hauser and running from forced chemotherapy treatments.
www.youtube.com/watch?v=qJimj5gs6cQ

Billy Best Speaks About Danny Hauser, Part 2

Mike Cann.net interviews Billy Best about Danny Hauser and running from forced chemotherapy treatments.
www.youtube.com/watch?v=ZPuKJEgLcJI

Cancer is a Fungus

Dr. Tullio Simoncini is an Italian doctor, specializing in oncology (cancer), diabetology and metabolic disorders. He believes every cancer begins with a fungus.
www.cancerisafungus.com

How to Prevent and Treat Cancer with Natural Medicine

Linda Devine recommends this book in interview about healing her breast cancer naturally.
www.thegoodwitch.ca/bookshelf/

Cauldron Shop

For copies of The Cancer Journal.
www.thegoodwitch.ca/cauldron_shop/

Cleanse Your Body ~ Download

Nine simple and very effective cleanses to help you start healing right away.
www.thegoodwitch.ca/start-with-cleanses-first/

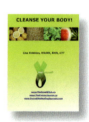

Cleanse ~ Cleansing Basics

An article on the basics of cleansing and what symptoms to look for when you are in need of cleansing or detoxing your body.
www.thegoodwitch.ca/cleansing-basics/

Doug Kaufmann's interview with Dr. Tullio Simoncini

Youtube video ~ Doug Kaufmann interviews Dr. Tullio Simoncini about Cancer, Fungus and Tumors. Lots of interesting stuff in this short video.
www.thegoodwitch.ca/cancer-is-a-fungus/

Dr. Gustavo Bounous

Dr. Bounous' extensive research in immune enhancement at McGill University.
www.immunotec.com/Dr._Gustavo_Bounous_Science_Specialist

Dr. Gustavo Bounous ~ Breakthrough In Cell-Defense

Dr. Bounous' years of research help you understand the importance of Glutathione production and precursor nutrients needed to boost immunity, health and vitality and protect your body against cancer, viruses, free radicals, bacteria, oxidation, toxins, poisons and radiation.
www.thegoodwitch.ca/bookshelf/

Dr. Duke's Phytochemical and Ethnobotanical Database

Query the database for chemicals and activities for thousands of plants.
www.ars-grin.gov/duke/

Eat

Simple ways to incorporate healing foods every day. Delicious recipes, tips and nutritional advice at TheGoodWitch.ca.
www.thegoodwitch.ca/category/nutrition/

Fats that Heal Fats that Kill

Udo Erasmus's unequalled resource and best-selling book.
www.thegoodwitch.ca/bookshelf/

FengSHe.org

Presenting balanced solutions ~ for individuals, groups, organizations and governments. FengSHe.org ~ A vital shift in principles, encouraging the nurturing feminine energy ~ for us, for our world.
www.fengshe.org/

Flax Oil As A True Aid Against Arthritis, Heart Infarction, Cancer and Other Diseases

The famous Budwig Flax Seed Oil and Protein diet, a scientific revolution connecting cancer and fat metabolism.
www.thegoodwitch.ca/bookshelf/

Flora

For product information only. The company does not sell Flor Essence herbal tea blend online, so you must go to a health food store.
www.florahealth.com

Food Diary ~ Your Complimentary Copy
Record your food choices and most importantly, how they make you feel! Make copies or print more directly from this link.
www.thegoodwitch.ca/food-diary/

Grail Spring's Holistic Detox
Madeleine Marentette, author and owner of Grail Springs tells her beautiful story of rejuvenation and healing in this wonderful book. With breathtaking photos, simple instructions and recipes for detoxification and cleansing from the award winning Grail Springs Body Mind Spirit Retreat and Spa ~ the next best thing to being there.
www.thegoodwitch.ca/bookshelf/

Greg Caton's Website
Food Technologist, Herbalist and Author Greg Caton has been incarcerated for selling *drugs* in the United States. Greg Caton manufactures and sells Cansema, the escharotic preparation that Pattie MacDonald used to cure four breast and two neck tumors.
www.gregcaton.com/

Greg Caton Escharotic Prep Part 1 of 3
In this video, Greg shows exactly how to prepare caustic medicines.
www.youtube.com/watch?v=9XaZlYbxGek

Greg Caton Escharotic Prep Part 2 of 3
www.youtube.com/watch?v=PmdstCSyDqs&NR=1

Greg Caton Escharotic Prep Part 3 of 3
www.youtube.com/watch?v=qgmQV5UgeDw&NR=1

Greg Caton's Meditopia
Greg Caton compiled evidence in his book *Meditopia*. You can read Chapters 1 to 6 at Meditopia.org.
www.meditopia.org/

Greg Caton kidnapped, deported by FDA ~ Natural News ~ Health Ranger Report #84
Mike Adams interviews Cathryn Caton. Free download of the mp3, look down the list to find the audio report in mp3 format.
www.naturalnews.com/Index-Podcasts.html

Healing Cancer From The Inside Out ~ Book

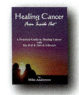

A book featuring testimonials of people who have cured themselves using *The Rave Diet*, a raw food diet.
www.thegoodwitch.ca/bookshelf/

Healing Cancer From The Inside Out ~ DVD

A documentary film, featuring testimonials of people who have cured themselves using a raw food diet.
www.thegoodwitch.ca/bookshelf/

Healing Cancer From The Inside Out ~ Trailer

Mariana Pina-Bergtold and Brenda Cobbs, talk about how they were pressured by doctors to have chemotherapy, radiation and surgery, but instead chose to heal themselves quickly and safely using raw foods.
www.youtube.com/v/
_xkyMAYmrQY&hl=en_US&fs=1&color1=0x402061&color2=0x9461ca

IARC Monographs

International Agency for Research on Cancer, Monographs on the Evaluation of Carcinogenic Risks to Humans.
www.monographs.iarc.fr/

Incredible Healing Journals

The Incredible Healing Journals ~ A community of people sharing true stories of healing naturally ~ Always streaming true stories of natural healing.
www.incrediblehealingjournals.com

Immunocal™ ~ Whey Protein Isolate

Patented natural health product with over ninety percent pure protein with a higher bioavailability than any other protein supplement available.
www.thegoodwitch.ca/cauldron_shop/

Jay Kordich ~ The Juice Daddy

Jay cured himself of bladder cancer at the age of 25. He lives on in excellent health, still promoting fresh juicing after all these years.
www.juicedaddy.com/

John Robbins ~ The New Good Life

The New Good Life motivates you to raise the quality of your health and life for more joy and true success.

www.thegoodwitch.ca/bookshelf/

John Robbins ~ Healthy At 100

John Robbins has compiled extensive information about the oldest and healthiest people on earth.

www.thegoodwitch.ca/bookshelf/

John Robbins ~ Diet For A New America

This book woke me up to the plight of animals that are affected by our way of living. It stirred every emotion with stories of courageous animals and their interactions with humans. John discusses the latest findings in nutritional research about our food choices and how they affect our health, happiness and future of life on earth. A timeless read.

www.thegoodwitch.ca/bookshelf/

John Robbins ~ Diet For A New America DVD

The DVD ~ How your food choices affect your health, happiness, and the future of life on earth.

www.thegoodwitch.ca/bookshelf/

Linda Devine's Interview Transcript

Transcript of my exclusive interview with Linda where she tells exactly how she healed from breast cancer in 10 months with diet and lifestyle changes.

www.thegoodwitch.ca/conversations-with-linda/

Linda Devine's Website

Linda is a dedicated healer who works endlessly to bring hope to others with joy, intelligence and enthusiasm.

www.lindadevine.com

Native American Ethonobotany database

This University of Michigan-Dearborn database holds: foods, drugs, dyes and fibers, derived from plants and used by Native Americans.

www.herb.umd.umich.edu/

Natural News

An unbiased network of empowering educational websites on natural health, offering thousands of articles, dozens of downloadable reports and guides, all free and without annoying pop-up ads.
www.naturalnews.com/Index.html

Neale Donald Walsch

The Complete Conversations with God ~ An unprecedented spiritual view with completely logical solutions to the problems in our lives and in our world.
www.thegoodwitch.ca/bookshelf/

North American Folk Healing

A Reader's Digest compilation from 1998. An excellent compilation of remedies used by native North Americans.
www.thegoodwitch.ca/bookshelf/

Nurse with Leukemia

Nurse tells her story to David Holland M.D. ~ She was diagnosed with Leukemia twice, but really had a fungal infection!
www.loveoffering.com/fungus.htm

Pattie MacDonald's Testimonial

Pattie's letter on the effectiveness of Cansema and how she used it to get rid of four breast and two neck tumors.
www.thegoodwitch.ca/breast-cancer-cured-with-escharotic/

pH Scale Of Common Foods ~ Your Complimentary Copy

Download a complimentary copy of pH Scale of Common Foods ~ print and stick to your refrigerator.
www.thegoodwitch.ca/ph-chart/

pH ~ Test your pH

Quick Instructions On How to test your pH at home.
www.thegoodwitch.ca/how-to-test-my-own-ph/

240

Pituitary Tumor on Raw Food Diet!

Kerri Howarth is an excellent teacher and an amazing raw food chef! In this interview, Kerri tells how she was diagnosed with a Pituitary Tumor and switched to a raw food diet to save her life . . . Interview in video, audio and transcript available to watch, listen to or read.
www.thegoodwitch.ca/pituitary

Skin Deep

Check the safety of your personal care products with the Cosmetics Safety Database.
http://www.ewg.org/skindeep/

Speakers From The Heart

Home to leading-edge thinkers, who inspire and teach others through their passion and honesty.
www.speakersfromtheheart.com/

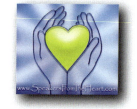

Stockholm Convention on Persistent Organic Pollutants

The Persistent Organic Pollutants Review Committee classifies persistent organic pollutants, lists worldwide inventories, and makes recommendations based on their research.
http://chm.pops.int/Convention/POPsReviewCommittee/hrPOPRCMeetings/POPRC2/AnnexFinformationYear2007/tabid/466/language/en-US/Default.aspx

Taber's Cyclopedic Medical Dictionary

Since 1940 ~ The definitive resource for definition of medical terms.
www.thegoodwitch.ca/bookshelf/

Tart Montmorency Cherry Concentrate

The superb Melatonin source.
www.thegoodwitch.ca/cauldron_shop/

The Acid Alkaline Food Guide

A Quick Reference to foods and their effect on the pH levels of your body. An excellent guide to controlling pH balance, improving your health and longevity.
www.thegoodwitch.ca/bookshelf/

The Biology Of Belief
Dr. Bruce Lipton shares a revolution in understanding about the ability of our thoughts to affect our lives and our health.
www.thegoodwitch.ca/bookshelf/

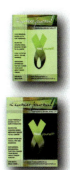

The Cancer Journal - Audio Version
For audio version of The Cancer Journal ~ Heal Yourself!
www.thegoodwitch.ca/cauldron_shop/

The Cancer Journal - Electronic Copy
For electronic copies of The Cancer Journal ~ Heal Yourself!
www.thegoodwitch.ca/cauldron_shop/

The Cancer Journal
For printed copies of The Cancer Journal ~ Heal Yourself!
www.thegoodwitch.ca/cauldron_shop/

The Complete Illustrated Holistic Herbal
Search *The Herbal* section by name of herb, identify herbs by photograph, look up symptoms, diseases or systems of your body.
www.thegoodwitch.ca/bookshelf/

The Complete Medicinal Herbal
A practical guide to the healing with detailed photographs and explicit directions for creating tinctures, infusions, decoctions, syrups, infused oils, creams, ointments, compresses and poultices.
www.thegoodwitch.ca/bookshelf/

The Essence of Essiac
Sheila Snow tells the story of Essiac, Rene Caisse's famous herbal cancer remedy. She used the remedy for over fifty years to heal thousands of cancer patients. Sheila researches several versions of the secret remedy and discloses essential information and detailed directions.
www.thegoodwitch.ca/bookshelf/

Forced Chemotherapy Daniel Hauser ~ 1
Mike Adams updates us on Daniel's situation and the issues surrounding the horrendous forced poisoning of one of America's children.
www.youtube.com/watch?v=pFNMM1bDDK8&feature=related

Forced Chemotherapy of Daniel Hauser ~ 2
Part Two ~ Mike Adams video commentary on Daniel Hauser.
www.youtube.com/watch?v=F84weZ6-Qu8&feature=related

The Good Witch

Heal Yourself! ~ Complimentary recipes,
simple cleanses, tips and tons of
information and resources on natural healing.
Free downloads, audios, videos ~ Motivation, Power, Truth!
www.thegoodwitch.ca/

The Green Pharmacy

From James Duke, considered to be the world's foremost authority on
healing herbs, and the author of Dr. Duke's *Phytochemical and
Ethnobotanical Database.*
www.thegoodwitch.ca/bookshelf/

The Macrobiotic Way

Founder of the *Kushi Institute* Michio Kushi's definitive guide to the
mostly widely accepted healing diet ~ Macrobiotic healing.
www.thegoodwitch.ca/bookshelf/

The Master Cleanser

Stanley Burrough's famous, simple lemonade, cayenne and maple syrup
cleanse ~ use cleansing to heal from any disease, detailed information.
www.thegoodwitch.ca/bookshelf/

The New Age Herbalist

A well rounded herbal resource with a glossary of herbs, sketches and
color photographs, body care, home care, relaxation, herbs for nutrition
and health, a large section on herbs for healing and information on
growing, cultivating, harvesting and storing herbs ~ useful recipes and
tips for culinary herbs, medicinal uses and making herbal steams, soaps,
lotions, shampoos, toothpaste and deodorant.
www.thegoodwitch.ca/bookshelf/

The New Optimum Nutrition Bible

Patrick Holford, leading expert, The New Optimum Nutrition Bible, "so
you can transform your life through optimum nutrition, to be free of pain
and full of health so you can enjoy your life to the full."
www.thegoodwitch.ca/bookshelf/

The Rave Diet & Lifestyle Book and DVD

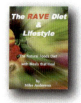

This book details the raw healing diet used by people who
were featured in the movie, *Healing Cancer From The
Inside Out.*
www.thegoodwitch.ca/bookshelf/

The Secret History Of The War On Cancer

If you really want to know why cancer rates continue to climb, you must read this book. An exhaustive resource of insights into why cancer is so prevalent today even though scientists and researchers have known for decades what actually causes it!
www.thegoodwitch.ca/bookshelf/

The Way Of Herbs

Complete, up to date information on simple herbal remedies for natural health and healing, with a revised chapter on botanical cancer treatments. Lots of recipes for experimenting with your own herbal blends.
www.thegoodwitch.ca/bookshelf/

Victoria Boutenko, The Raw Family ~ Fresh

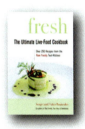

Fresh, I love, love, love this book! Victoria is considered the *guru* of green smoothies and going raw. My favorite raw food chefs, The Raw Family.
www.thegoodwitch.ca/bookshelf/

When Healing Becomes A Crime

When Healing Becomes A Crime, The Amazing Story of the Hoxsey Cancer Clinics and the Return of Alternative Therapies.
www.thegoodwitch.ca/bookshelf/

Women's Health Initiative

A massive, 15 year study definitively proved the link between synthetic hormones like those in hormone replacement therapy and birth control and reproductive cancers, especially breast cancer. The study also proved risks for heart disease, stroke and blood clots.
www.nhlbi.nih.gov/whi/

World Without Cancer

Edward G. Griffin exposes the truth about suppression of natural cancer cures in this amazing story about B17 deficiency and its link to cancer.
www.thegoodwitch.ca/bookshelf/

Yoga Mastering The Basics

A large, beautiful and well illustrated yoga masterpiece.
www.thegoodwitch.ca/bookshelf/

Yvonne Chamberlain ~ Why Me, Kicking Cancer and Other Life Changing Stuff

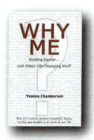

Yvonne teaches simply and eloquently how to overcome your previous thought patterns and change your core beliefs to heal from one of the most deadly diseases.
www.whyme.net.au/Buy-Why-Me.html

Yvonne Chamberlain's Interview MP3 and Transcript

Hear my exclusive interview with Yvonne who diagnosed with deadly black melanoma, given only 6 weeks to live, and facing amputation of her leg. She took control, refused to believe her doctor's dire predictions and is here to tell her story 28 years later with both her legs and a 28 years of cancer freedom.
www.thegoodwitch.ca/yvonne-takes-on-black-melanoma/

Yvonne Chamberlain's Website

WhyMe.net.au ~ Sign up for Yvonne's fortnightly newsletters.
www.WhyMe.net.au

Affiliate Disclosure

Some of the links in this book are to books and products I have an affiliation with. I have chosen these affiliations because their information, products and services may be of tremendous benefit if you decide that is what will help you at this time. I wrote about them in this book because *I know they can help you!* You can see affiliate id's inside some of the links. This income helps pay for costs associated with my work. If you choose to click on a link and purchase a product I may get a small commission for guiding you to that resource. If you wish to learn more about affiliate income, I suggest you visit
www.WonderfulWebWomen.com (p.s. men are very welcome too!)

References

If you cannot link to a reference it is possible the reference may have been moved. Wherever possible, I have kept copies of these documents in the case their website address has been changed, and so have proof should they ever be deleted or moved from their present url.

Adam (2010) *Intention Heals Research Projects (Mind Over Matter)*. Accessed October 27, 2010 from http://www.intentionheals.com/

Adam Dreamhealer (2010) *About Adam*. Dreamhealer.com. Accessed October 27, 2010 from http://www.dreamhealer.com/about

Adams, Mike. (2009) *Daniel Hauser and the Side Effects of Cancer Treatments for Hodgkin's Disease*. NaturalNews.com. Retrieved October 21, 2010 from http://www.naturalnews.com/026386_cancer_radiation_treatment.html

Adams, Mike. (2009) FDA dupes Interpol to achieve illegal kidnapping and deportation of herbal formulator Greg Caton. Accessed November 8, 2010 from http://www.naturalnews.com/027750_Greg_Caton_FDA.html

Adams, Mike. (2010) Free Greg Caton from FDA tyranny; your help needed. Accessed November 8, 2010 from http://www.naturalnews.com/028306_Greg_Caton_FDA.html

American Cancer Society. (2007) *Cancer Facts & Figures - 2007*. PDF Obtained October 29, 2010 from http://www.cancer.org/Research/CancerFactsFigures/cancer-facts-figures-2007

American Cancer Society. (2009) *Second Cancers Caused By Cancer Treatment*. Retrieved October 16, 2010 from http://www.cancer.org/Cancer/CancerCauses/OtherCarcinogens/MedicalTreatments/SecondCancersCausedbyCancerTreatment/second-cancers-caused-by-cancer-treatment-treatments-linked-to-second-cancers

Anderson, Sandra. & Sovik, Rolf. (2000) *Yoga Mastering the Basics*. Pennsylvania: Himalayan Institute Press.

Angell, Marcia. (2004) *Excess in the pharmaceutical industry*. Canadian Medical Association Journal. Retrieved October 21, 2010 from http://www.cmaj.ca/cgi/content/full/171/12/1451

AstraZeneca. (2009) *AstraZeneca PLC Fourth Quarter and Full Year Results 2008*. PDF obtained October 21, 2010 from http://www.astrazeneca.com/media/latest-press-releases/2009/AZN-Q4-Results?itemId=4759388

AstraZeneca. (2010) *Work at Alderley Park, Cheshire. Astra Zeneca United Kingdom*. Retrieved October 20, 2010 from http://ideas.astrazeneca.com/our-locations/alderley-park/work-at-Alderley-Park?itemId=4231693&nav=yes (Inactive link).

246

AstraZeneca United Kingdom. (2010) *Ten year data confirm combination of early and long-term advantage of ARIMIDEX (anastrozole) over tamoxifen.* AstraZeneca United Kingdom Graduate Careers. Retrieved October 20, 2010 from http://www.astrazeneca.co.uk/search/?itemId=10945728

AstraZeneca Canada Ltd. (2010) *Product Monograph, Nolvadex-D, Tamoxifen Citrate.* PDF obtained October 20, 2010 from http://www.astrazeneca.ca/documents/ProductPortfolio/NOLVADEX_PM_en.pdf

Ausubel, Kenny. (2000) *When Healing Becomes A Crime.* Vermont: Healing Arts Press.

Ballentine, M.D., Rudolph. (1978) *Diet & Nutrition: A Holistic Approach.* Pennsylvania: The Himalayan International Institute.

BBC News Online. 1 (2008, November 12) *Doctors 'rely on chemo too much'.* Retrieved October 21, 2010 from http://news.bbc.co.uk/2/hi/health/7722626.stm

BBC News Online. 2 (2008, April 22) *Brain damage link to cancer drug.* Retrieved October 21, 2010 from http://news.bbc.co.uk/2/hi/health/7360127.stm

Berry, Drew. (2006) *Apoptosis and Signal Transduction.* Accessed November 9, 2010 from http://www.wehi.edu.au/education/wehitv/apoptosis_and_signal_transduction/

Best, Bill & Best, Sue. (2010) *Billy's Story.* Accessed October 27, 2010 from http://www.billybest.net/BillysStory.htm

Bowden, Jonny. (2007) *The 150 Healthiest Foods on Earth.* Massachusetts: Fair Winds Press.

Brenner, David J., Hall, Eric J., Phil, D. (2007) *Computed Tomography - An Increasing Source of Radiation Exposure.* Retrieved October 16, 2010 from The New England Journal of Medicine online at http://www.nejm.org/doi/full/10.1056/NEJMra072149

Bois, P. (1964) *Tumour of the Thymus in Magnesium-deficient Rats.* Nature. Abstract obtained from http://www.nature.com/nature/journal/v204/n4965/abs/2041316a0.html

Brown, Dana. (2008) *Sick boy's family in court today.* TheStar.com. Retrieved October 21, 2010 from http://www.thestar.com/article/424747

Brown, Susan., & Trivieri, Larry. (2006) *The Acid Alkaline Food Guide.* New York: Square One Publishers.

Buchman, Dian Dincin. (1996) *Herbal Medicine: The Natural Way to Get Well and Stay Well.* New York: Wings Books.

Budwig, Johanna. (1994) *Flax Oil As A True Aid Against Arthritis, Heart Infarction, Cancer And Other Diseases*. British Columbia: Apple Publishing Company Ltd.

Canadian Cancer Society. (2010) *Annual Report 2009/2010*. Retrieved October 16, 2010 from http://annualreport.cancer.ca/

Canadian Cancer Society Research Institute. (2010) *The Canadian Cancer Society Research Institute*. Retrieved October 16, 2010 from http://www.cancer.ca/Canada-wide/Cancer%20research/Funding%20cancer%20research/Role%20of%20the%20Canadian%20Cancer%20Society%20Research%20Institute.aspx?sc_lang=en

Canada Revenue Agency. (2010) *Schedule 6: Detailed Financial Information - CANADIAN CANCER SOCIETY (NOVA SCOTIA DIVISION)*. Retrieved October 16, 2010 from http://www.cra-arc.gc.ca/ebci/haip/srch/t3010form21sched6-eng.action?b=118829803RR0006&e=2009-01-31&n=CANADIAN+CANCER+SOCIETY+ONTARIO+DIVISION&r=http%3A%2F%2Fwww.cra-arc.gc.ca%3A80%2Febci%2Fhaip%2Fsrch%2Ft3010form21-eng.action%3Fb%3D118829803RR0006%26amp%3Be%3D2009-01-31%26amp%3Bn%3DCANADIAN%2BCANCER%2BSOCIETY%2BONTARIO%2BDIVISION%26amp%3Br%3Dhttp%253A%252F%252Fwww.cra-arc.gc.ca%253A80%252Febci%252Fhaip%252Fsrch%252Fbasicsearchresult-eng.action%253Fs%253Dregistered%2526amp%253Bk%253DCanadian%252BCancer%252BSociety%2526amp%253Bp%253D1%2526amp%253Bb%253Dtrue

Cardis, Elisabeth., Kesminiene, Ausrele., Ivanov, Victor., Malakhova, Irina., Shibata, Yoshisada., Khrouch, Valeryi., et al. (2005) *Risk of Thyroid Cancer After Exposure to 131Iodine in Childhood. Journal of the National Cancer Institute*. Abstract obtained October 25, 2010 from http://jnci.oxfordjournals.org/content/97/10/724.full?ijkey=78i7V4IS1XnJ5v0&keytype=ref

Carthew, P., Martin, E.A., White, I.N.H., De Matteis, F., Edwärds, RE., Dorman, et al. (1995) *Tamoxifen induces short-term cumulative DNA damage and liver tumors in rats: promotion by phenobarbital*. Cancer Res., 55, 544-547. PDF obtained from http://cancerres.aacrjournals.org/search?fulltext=tamoxifen+induces+short&submit=yes&x=9&y=11

Caton, Greg. (2006) Meditopia. Obtained November 8, 2010 from http://www.meditopia.org/index_ing.htm

Caton, Greg. (2009) Escharotic Preparations - Intro by Greg Caton, Part 1 of 3. Accessed November 8, 2010 from http://www.youtube.com/watch?v=9XaZlYbxGek

Caton, Greg. (2009) Escharotic Preparations - Intro by Greg Caton, Part 2 of 3. Accessed November 8, 2010 from http://www.youtube.com/watch?v=PmdstCSyDqs&NR=1

Caton, Greg. (2009) Escharotic Preparations - Intro by Greg Caton, Part 3 of 3. Accessed November 8, 2010 from http://www.youtube.com/watch?v=qgmQV5UgeDw&NR=1

Choi, B.T., Choeng, J., Choi, Y.H. (2003) *Beta-Lapachone-induced apoptosis is associated with activation of caspase-3 and inactivation of NF-kappaB in human colon cancer HCT-116 cells.* PubMed.gov. Abstract obtained October 25, 2010 from http://www.ncbi.nlm.nih.gov/pubmed/14597880? ordinalpos=1&itool=EntrezSystem2.PEntrez.Pubmed.Pubmed_ResultsPanel.Pu bmed_SingleItemSupl.Pubmed_Discovery_RA&linkpos=3&log $=relatedarticles&logdbfrom=pubmed

Christiansen, Cindy L., Wang, Fei., Barton, Mary B., Kreuter, William., Elmore, Joann G., Gelfand, Alan E., et al. (2000) *Predicting the Cumulative Risk of False-Positive Mammograms.* Abstract obtained from http:// jnci.oxfordjournals.org/content/92/20/1657.full? maxtoshow=&HITS=10&hits=10&RESULTFORMAT=1&author1=Christiansen %25252C+Cindy +&andorexacttitle=and&andorexacttitleabs=and&andorexactfulltext=and&searc hid=1&FIRSTINDEX=0&sortspec=relevance&volume=92&resourcetype=HWCI T

Church & Dwight Co., Inc. (2008) *Will ARM & HAMMER® Baking Soda work as an antacid?* Retrieved October 18, 2010 from http://www.armhammer.com/ basics/magic/#12

Cousens, M.D., Gabriel. (2010) *Juice Fast For Peace.* Retrieved October 15, 2010 from http://www.juicefastforpeace.com/

Davis, Devra. (2007) The Secret History of the War on Cancer. New York: Basic Books.

Day, Phillip. (1999) *Why We're Still Dying To Know The Truth.* United Kingdom: Credence Publications.

DeNoon, Daniel J. (2003) *Hormone Melatonin Slows Breast Cancer. David E. Blask's speech at annual meeting of American Association for Cancer Research. WebMD Breast Cancer Health Center.* Accessed November 1, 2010 from http:// www.webmd.com/breast-cancer/news/20030714/hormone-melatonin-slows-breast-cancer

Dr. Duke's *Phytochemical and Ethnobotanical Database.* (1998) *Specific Queries of the Phytochemical Database.* Retrieved October 21, 2010 from http:// www.ars-grin.gov/duke/

Duke, James A. (1997) *The Green Pharmacy.* Pennsylvania: Rodale Press.

Erasmus, Udo. (1993) *Fats That Heal, Fats That Kill.* British Columbia: Alive Books.

Esko, Wendy. (1978) *Introducing Macrobiotic Cooking.* Tokyo: Japan Publications.

Fahey, Jed W., Zhang, Yuesheng., Talalay, Paul. Broccoli sprouts: An exceptionally rich source of inducers of enzymes that protect against chemical carcinogens. PNAS Vol. 94 No. 19 10367-10372, September 16, 1997. The National Academy of Sciences of the USA. Retrieved February 8, 2011 from http://www.pnas.org/content/94/19/10367.full.pdf

Flora Essence. (2010) *Herbal Blends.* Accessed October 25, 2010 from http://www.florahealth.com/flora/home/Canada/Products/R8070.htm

Griffin, Edward G. (1974) *A World Without Cancer.* Youtube.com. Accessed October 27, 2010 from http://www.youtube.com/watch?v=NQMf8NnJo7Q&feature=related
Somersall, Dr. Allan C. & Bounous, Dr. Gustavo. (2001) *Breakthrough in Cell-Defense: How to Benefit from the REAL Glutathione Revolution.* Toronto: GoldenEight Publishers.

Griffin, Edward G. (1996) *World Without Cancer.* California: American Media.

Griggs, Barbara. (1994) *The Green Witch Herbal.* Vermont: Healing Arts Press

Hardeland, Rüdiger., & Poeggeler, Burkhard. (2003) *Non-vertebrate melatonin. Melatonin in food and medicinal plants.* PDF obtained November 1, 2010 from http://onlinelibrary.wiley.com/doi/10.1034/j.1600-079X.2003.00040.x/full
Hardeland, Rüdiger & Pandi-Perumal, S.R. (2005) *Melatonin, a potent agent in antioxidative defense: Actions as a natural food constituent, gastrointestinal factor, drug and prodrug.* Nutrition & Metabolism (Table 2) Accessed November 1, 2010 from http://www.dietaryfiberfood.com/melatonin-natural-sources.php

Hartwell, Jonathan. (1984) *Plants Used Against Cancer A Survey.* Massachusetts: Quarterman Publications.

Hattori, A., Migitaki, H., Iigo, M., Itoh, M., Yamamoto, K., Ohtani-Kaneko, R., Hara, M., Suzuki, T., Reiter, R.J. (1995) *Identification of melatonin in plants and its effects on plasma melatonin levels and binding to melatonin receptors in vertebrates.* Publication details accessed November 1, 2010 from http://www.researchgate.net/publication/15426392_Identification_of_melatonin_in_plants_and_its_effects_on_plasma_melatonin_levels_and_binding_to_melatonin_receptors_in_vertebrates

Health Canada. (2007) *Mammography. It's Your Health.* Retrieved October 20, 2010 from http://www.hc-sc.gc.ca/hl-vs/iyh-vsv/med/mammog-eng.php

Hill, Steven M., & Blask, David E. (1988) *Effects of the Pineal Hormone Melatonin on the Proliferation and Morphological Characteristics of Human Breast Cancer Cells (MCF-7) in Culture.* American Association for Cancer Research. Abstract obtained November 1, 2010 from http://cancerres.aacrjournals.org/content/48/21/6121.abstract

Hoffman, David. (1996) *The Complete Illustrated Holistic Herbal.* Dorset: Element Books Limited.

Holford, Patrick. (2004) *The New Optimum Nutrition Bible.* California: The Crossing Press.

Holland, David. (2010) *Nurse with leukaemia treated with antifungals.* Retrieved October 18, 2010 from http://www.loveoffering.com/fungus.htm

Hong, Xin-Yu., Chou, Yu-Cheng., Lazareff, Jorge A. (2008) *Brain stem candidiasis mimicking cerebellopontine angle tumor.* Surgical Neurology. Abstract obtained on October 18, 2010 from http://www.surgicalneurology-online.com/article/S0090-3019%2808%2900009-8/abstract

Hoxsey, Harry. (1957) *You Don't Have To Die.* New York: Milestone Books.

Huang, Qing. (2007) *Anti-cancer properties of anthraquinones from rhubarb.* PubMed.gov. Abstract obtained October 25, 2010 from http://www.ncbi.nlm.nih.gov/pubmed/17022020

Hunt, Barbara J., Belanger, Leonard F. (1972) *Localized, multiform, sub-periosteal hyperplasia and generalized osteomyelosclerosis in magnesium-deficient rats.* SpringerLink. Abstract obtained October 21, 2010 from http://www.springerlink.com/content/j77201862q92q162/

IARC, International Agency For Research On Cancer. (2010) *IARC Monographs on the Evaluation of Carcinogenic Risks to Humans.* IARC Monograph on Tamoxifen. PDF obtained on October 20, 2010 from http://monographs.iarc.fr/cgi-bin/htsearch

Immunotec. (2010) Patents. Accessed October 27. 2010 from http://www.immunotec.com/IRL/Public/en/CAN/science_patents.wcp?&site=LISA265999
Iriti, Marcello., Varoni, Elena M., Vitalini, Sara. (2010) *Melatonin in traditional Mediterranean diets.* (Abstract obtained November 1, 2010 from http://onlinelibrary.wiley.com/doi/10.1111/j.1600-079X.2010.00777.x/full

Kollewe, Julia & Wearden, Graeme. (2007) *ICI: from Perspex to paints.* Guardian.co.uk. Retrieved October 20, 2010 from http://www.guardian.co.uk/business/2007/jun/18/2

Kim, S.O., Kwon, J.I., Jeong, Y.K., Kim, G.Y., Kim, N.D., Choi, Y.H. (2007) *Induction of Egr-1 is associated with anti-metastatic and anti-invasive ability of beta-lapachone in human hepatocarcinoma cells.* PubMed.gov. Abstract obtained October 25, 2010 from http://www.ncbi.nlm.nih.gov/pubmed/17827686?dopt=Citation

Kushi, Michio. (2004) *The Macrobiotic Way, The Definitive Guide To Macrobiotic Living.* New York: Penguin Group (USA) Inc.

Lamm, Donald., & Riggs, Dale, R. (2001) *Enhanced Immunocompetence by Garlic: Role in Bladder Cancer and Other Malignancies.* The Journal of Nutrition. Abstract obtained October 27, 2010 from http://jn.nutrition.org/cgi/content/abstract/131/3/1067S

Lee, Christoph I., Haims, Andrew H., Monico, Edward P., Brink, James A., Forman, Howard P. (2004) *Diagnostic CT Scans: Assessment of Patient, Physician and Radiologist Awareness of Radiation Dose and Possible Risks.* Journal Radiology. 2004 Mar:18: 231, 393-398. PDF retrieved October 18, 2010 at Radiology online from http://radiology.rsna.org/content/231/2/393.abstract

Levin, Allen. (1990) *The Healing Of Cancer.* San Francisco: 1990.

Li, Dr. William. (2010) *William Li: Can We Eat To Starve Cancer? Ted: Ideas Worth Spreading.* Accessed October 27, 2010 from http://www.ted.com/talks/william_li.html

Lipton, Bruce. (2009) *The Biology Of Belief.* New York: Hay House Inc.

Lissoni, Paolo., Rovelli, Franco., Malugani, Fabio., Bucovec, Roberta., Conti, Ario., Maestroni, Georges J.M. (2001) *Anti-angiogenic activity of melatonin in advanced cancer patients.* Obtained November 1, 2010 from http://www.nel.edu/22_1/NEL220101A05_Lissoni__.pdf

Living Well With Cancer Information Centre. (2001) *Living Well With Cancer, From Effects of Cancer and Treatment,* Healthy Eating brochure. Retrieved October 15, 2010 from http://www.livingwellwithcancer.com/english/pdfs/HCPguide_ENG.pdf

Marquart, Karl-Horst. (2006) *Electron microscopy reveals fungal cells within tumor tissue from two African patients with AIDS-associated Kaposi sarcoma.* Ultrastructural Pathology. Abstract obtained October 18, 2010 from http://www.ncbi.nlm.nih.gov/pubmed/16825120

Mabey, Richard., (1988) *The New Age Herbalist.* New York: Collier Books.

Marentette, Madeleine. (2007) Grail Springs Holistic Detox for Body, Mind & Spirit. Toronto: McArthur & Company.

Marieb, Elaine N. (2003) *Essentials of Human Anatomy & Physiology.* Seventh Edition. California: Pearson Education Inc., publishing as Benjamin Cummings.

McGill University Newsroom. (2010) Low levels of Vitamin D linked to muscle fat, decreased strength in young people. Accessed November 8, 2010 from http://www.mcgill.ca/newsroom/news/item/?item_id=115221

MDS Inc. 1 (2008, June) *I-123 Fact Sheet, Iodine-123 Radiochemical Sodium Iodide Solution.* Retrieved October 18, 2010 from http://www.mdsnordion.com/documents/products/I-123_Solu_Bel.pdf (Inactive Link). New Link: http://www.nordion.com/our_products/molecular_medicine_products.asp. October 13, 2011.

MDS Inc. 2 (2008) *MDS Inc. Annual Information Form for the year ended October 31, 2007.* Retrieved October 18, 2010 from http://www.mdsnordion.com/reports/2007_engaif.pdf .

Mettler, F.A. Jr., Wiest, P.W., Locken, J.A., Kelsey, C.A. (2000) *CT Scanning: patterns of use and dose.* Journal Radiology Prot. 2000 Dec;20(4):353:9. Abstract obtained October 18, 2010 at PubMed.gov from http://www.ncbi.nlm.nih.gov/pubmed/11140709?dopt=Abstract

Miller, A.B., To, T., Baines, C.J., Wall, C. (2002) *The Canadian National Breast Screening Study-1: breast cancer mortality after 11 to 16 years follow-up. A randomized screening trial of mammography in women age 40 to 49 years.* Abstract obtained October 21, 2010 from http://www.ncbi.nlm.nih.gov/pubmed/12204013

National Breast Cancer Awareness Month. (2010) *Disease Information |
Mammogram Screening*. Retrieved October 21, 2010 from http://
www.nbcam.org/disease_mammogram_screening.cfm

National Cancer Institute. (2007) *Can Radiation Therapy Influence the
Development of Second Cancers?* Retrieved October 16, 2010 from http://
benchmarks.cancer.gov/2007/01/can-radiation-therapy-influence-the-
development-of-second-cancers/

National Cancer Institute. (2010) *Fact Sheet, Screening Mammograms*.
Retrieved October 21, 2010 from http://www.cancer.gov/cancertopics/factsheet/
detection/screening-mammograms

NaturalNews.com (2010) Health Ranger Report #84: Greg Caton kidnapped,
deported by FDA. Accessed November 8, 2010 from http://
www.naturalnews.com/Index-Podcasts.html

NBCAM. (2010) *National Breast Cancer Awareness Month, About Us, About
NBCAM*. Retrieved October 20, 2010 from http://www.nbcam.org/
about_nbcam.cfm

Ody, Penelope. (1993) *The Complete Medicinal Herbal*. London: Dorling
Kindersley Limited.

Ontario Ministry of Agriculture. (2003) *Ontario Weeds: Common Barberry*.
Food & Rural Affairs. Retrieved October 21, 2010 from http://
www.omafra.gov.on.ca/english/crops/facts/ontweeds/common_barberry.htm

Perera, Judith. (1985) *How chemical companies rose to the challenge*. New
Scientist. Retrieved October 20, 2010 from http://books.google.ca/books?
id=q7v_rDKouOgC&pg=PA36&lpg=PA36&dq=agent+orange
+ici&source=bl&ots=H9LoQTBPEK&sig=xwG119rcK0-
bnyRRcK0y8LUsBWE&hl=en&ei=TBW_TMSSIImknQeu7NWJDg&sa=X&oi=bo
ok_result&ct=result&resnum=7&ved=0CDQQ6AEwBg#v=onepage&q=agent
%20orange%20ici&f=false

Perrault, Danielle. (2001) *Nutritional Symptomatology*. Richmond Hill,
Ontario: CSNN Publishing.

Radiological Society of North America, Inc. (2010) *Patient Safety: Radiation
Exposure in X-ray and CT Examinations*. Retrieved October 18, 2010 from
http://www.radiologyinfo.org/en/safety/index.cfm?pg=sfty_xray#part2

Reader's Digest. (1998) *North American Folk Healing*. New York: The Reader's
Digest Association, Inc.

Reiter, Russel J. & Tan, Dan-Xian. (2002) *Melatonin: An antioxidant in edible
plants. Ann. N. Y. Acad. Sci. (Table 1)* Accessed November 1, 2010 from http://
www.dietaryfiberfood.com/melatonin-natural-sources.php

Reuters Health Information, (2010) *U.S. Prescription Drug Sales Hit $300
Billion in 2009*. Retrieved October 16, 2010 from http://www.reuters.com/
article/idUSTRE6303CU20100401

Robbins, John. (1987) *Diet For A New America*. California: H.J. Kramer.

Robbins, John. (2006) *Healthy At 100: How You Can At Any Age Dramatically Increase Your Life Span And Your Health Span*. New York: Random House.

Robey, Ian. F., Baggett, Brenda K., Kirkpatrick, Nathaniel D., Roe, Denise J., Dosescu, Julie., Sloane, Bonnie F., et al. (2009) *Bicarbonate Increases Tumor pH and Inhibits Spontaneous Metastases*. Retrieved October 18, 2010 from http://cancerres.aacrjournals.org/content/69/6/2260.long

Saul, Andrew W. (2007) *Topical Vitamin C Stops Basal Cell Carcinoma*. Orthomolecular.org. Accessed October 27, 2010 from http://www.orthomolecular.org/resources/omns/v03n12.shtml

Securities and Exchange Commission. (2005) *Transition Report Pursuant to Section 13 or 15(d) of the Securities Exchange Act of 1934, Commission file number: 1-15152, Syngenta AG, Switzerland*. Retrieved October 20, 2010 from http://yahoo.brand.edgar-online.com/EFX_dll/EDGARpro.dll?FetchFilingHTML1?ID=3543832&SessionID=l2R1HqxOZWHyxz7

Sharman, Edward H., Sharman, Kahzhl G., Bondy, Stephen C. (2010) *Extended exposure to dietary melatonin reduces tumour number and size in aged male mice*. PubMed.gov. Abstract obtained November 1, 2010 from http://www.ncbi.nlm.nih.gov/pubmed/20837128

Sircus, Mark. (2010) *Magnesium and Cancer Research*. *MagnesiumForLife.com*. Retrieved October 21, 2010 from http://magnesiumforlife.com/medical-application/magnesium-and-cancer/

Skin Deep Cosmetic Safety Database. (2010) *Sunsilk Hairapy Captivating Curls De-Frizz Leave-In Cream*. Accessed November 8, 2010 from http://www.ewg.org/skindeep/product/174363/Sunsilk_Hairapy_Captivating_Curls_De-Frizz_Conditioner/ (Modified Link).

Snow, Sheila. (1996) *The Essence of Essiac*. Canada: Self published.

Spangler, Luita D. (1996) *Xenoestrogens and Breast Cancer: Nowhere to Run*. Accessed November 1, 2010 from http://www.lindane.org/health/toxicology/breast_cancer.htm#risks

Springer-Verlag. (2002) *Session I: Helical CT and Cancer Risk, Panel Discussion*. PDF obtained October 21, 2010 from http://www.springerlink.com/content/p1wwgcyddu2wqrjy/

Staton, Tracy., Martino, Maureen. (2008) *Top 17 Paychecks in Big Pharma*. Fierce Pharma. Retrieved October 21, 2010 from http://www.fiercepharma.com/special-reports/top-17-paychecks-big-pharma

Stockholm Convention on Persistent Organic Pollutants (2007) *Lindane*. Accessed November 1, 2010 from http://chm.pops.int/Convention/POPsReviewCommittee/hrPOPRCMeetings/POPRC2/AnnexFinformationYear2007/tabid/466/language/en-US/Default.aspx

Sutton, Rebecca. (2008) Teen Girls' Body Burden of Hormone Altering Cosmetics Chemicals: Adolescent exposures to cosmetic chemicals of concern. Environmental Working Group. Accessed November 8, 2010 from http://www.ewg.org/reports/teens

Szabo, Liz. (2009, December 14). *Radiation from CT scans linked to cancers, deaths.* USA Today online. Retrieved October 18, 2010, from http://www.usatoday.com/news/health/2009-12-15-radiation15_st_N.htm

Terman, Michael & Terman, Jiuan Su. (2007) *Treatment of Seasonal Affective Disorder with a High-Output Negative Ionizer.* The Journal of Alternative and Complementary Medicine. Obtained November 10, 2010 from http://www.liebertonline.com/doi/abs/10.1089/acm.1995.1.87

TheHealthRanger. 1 (2009) *Health Freedom and the forced chemotherapy of Daniel Hauser.* YouTube.com. Accessed October 21, 2010 from http://www.youtube.com/watch?v=pFNMM1bDDK8&p=4AE732D1A4B2F9BA&playnext=1&index=1

TheHealthRanger. 2 (2009) *The forced chemotherapy of Daniel Hauser (part two).* YouTube.com. Accessed October 21, 2010 from http://www.youtube.com/watch?v=F84weZ6-Qu8&feature=related

The Angiogenesis Foundation. (2010) *Find Cancer Fighting Foods. Eat To Defeat Cancer.* Article accessed October 25, 2010 from http://www.eattodefeat.org/foods.php

The State of Israel, Ministry of Health. (2003) *MDS Nordion S.A. Kit for Preparation of Technetium Medronate Injection.* Retrieved October 18, 2010 from http://www.health.gov.il/units/pharmacy/trufot/alonim/822.pdf

Tierra, Michael. (1998) *The Way Of Herbs.* New York: Pocket Books.

Tobe, John H. (1977) *The Miracle of Live Juices and Raw Foods.* St. Catherines, Ontario: Provoker Press.

Trowbridge, John Parks., Walker, Morton. (1986) *The Yeast Syndrome.*

University of California, Riverside. (2000) *About Vitamin D.* Accessed November 9, 2010 from http://vitamind.ucr.edu/about.html

University of Granada (2007) *High Melatonin Content Can Help Delay Aging, Mouse Study Suggests.* ScienceDaily. Accessed November 1, 2010 from http://www.sciencedaily.com/releases/2007/04/070424062819.htm

University of Michigan-Dearborn. (2010) *Native American Ethnobotany, A Database of Foods, Drugs, Dyes and Fibers of Native American Peoples, Derived from Plants.* Accessed October 25, 2010 from http://herb.umd.umich.edu/

U.S. Preventive Services Task Force. (2009) *Screening for Breast Cancer.* Retrieved October 21, 2010 from http://www.uspreventiveservicestaskforce.org/uspstf/uspsbrca.htm

Venes, Donald & Thomas, Clayton L. (Eds.). (2001) *Taber's Cyclopedic Medical Dictionary*. Philadelphia: F.A. Davis Company.

Vogel, Virgil J. (1970) *American Indian Medicine*. Oklahoma: University of Oklahoma Press.

Voner, Valerie. (2003) *The Everything Reflexology Book. Manipulate zones in the hands and feet to relieve stress, improve circulation, and promote good health*. Maryland: Adams Media Corporation.

Waldron, H.A. (1983) *A brief history of scrotal cancer*. Obtained November 1, 2010 from http://www.ncbi.nlm.nih.gov/pmc/articles/PMC1009212/pdf/brjindmed00056-0030.pdf

Wallenborn, White McKenzie. (1997) *George Washington's Terminal Illness: A Modern Medical Analysis of the Last Illness and Death of George Washington. The Papers of George Washington, Articles*. Retrieved on October 21, 2010 from http://gwpapers.virginia.edu/articles/wallenborn.html

Warburg, Otto. (1931) *Nobel Lecture: The Oxygen-Transferring Ferment of Respiration*. Nobelprize.org. Obtained October 27, 2010 from http://nobelprize.org/nobel_prizes/medicine/laureates/1931/warburg-lecture.html

Warburg, Otto. (1969) *The Prime Cause and Prevention of Cancer - Part 1. Revised lecture at the meeting of the Nobel-Laureates at Lindau, Lake Constance, Germany. English Edition by Dean Burk, National Cancer Institute, Bethesda, Maryland, USA. The Second Revised Edition Published by Konrad Triltsch, Würzburg, Germany*. Accessed October 27, 2010 from http://healingtools.tripod.com/primecause1.html/primecause2.html

Wasserman, Scott. (2010) *Daniel Hauser Turns 14, Is Cancer Free*. Retrieved October 21, 2010 from http://www.myfoxtwincities.com/dpp/news/Daniel-Hauser-Turns-14,-Is-Cnacer-Free-mar-28-2010

Weinberg, Robert. A. (1998) *One Renegade Cell*. The Science Masters Series. New York: Basic Books.

Women's Health Initiative. (2010) *Women's Health Initiative*. Department of Health and Human Services. National Institutes of Health. National Heart, Lung, and Blood Institute. Accessed November 8, 2010 from http://www.nhlbi.nih.gov/whi/

World Cancer Research Fund. (2007) *Food, Nutrition, Physical Activity, and the Prevention of Cancer: a Global Perspective - Online*. Retrieved October 15, 2010, from http://www.dietandcancerreport.org/

About The Author

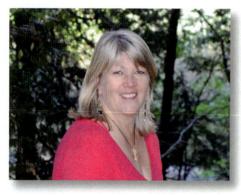

Lisa Robbins, BScHN, RHN, CTT, is a Registered Holistic Nutritionist with an honors degree of Bachelor of Science in Holistic Nutrition.

Lisa is a passionate teacher, author, interviewer and public speaker.

Lisa lives in the beautiful rolling hills of rural Southern Ontario. Her backyard is a forest of evergreens and maple trees, deer, rabbits and coywolves.

When Lisa isn't in her kitchen experimenting with and blending herbal remedies, you'll find her in her large organic garden tending to a bountiful harvest of native medicinal and culinary herbs, flowers and vegetables.

Lisa lives with Bob, her husband of 26 years. They have three beautiful children Alix, Luke and Anna and live with Ashley, a beautiful and neurotic dog, the odd stray cat and *way too many plants*!

Lisa's other hobbies include photography, videography, web design, sports and yoga.

On The Web

www.TheGoodWitch.ca

Delicious healing recipes, tips, information and connection to hundreds of unbiased resources for healing; studies, journal articles, resource databases, books, audios and videos, many free. Successful healing stories in videos, audios, transcripts of interviews and articles all about healing naturally. Enter your name and email to receive notification when new recipes, cleanses, articles, interviews and free downloads are available.

www.IncredibleHealingJournals.com

The Incredible Healing Journals ~ a truly alternative healing community ~ find incredible stories of natural healing streaming through our front page. Connect with natural healers and their own stories of healing, tips, advice and support.

www.HealingCancer.ca

All about Healing Cancer ~ resources, lessons, interviews, videos, audios, incredible healing stories, articles, truth and empowerment!

16405034R00144

Made in the USA
Charleston, SC
18 December 2012